T0210253

Management of Endocrine Tumors

Editor

NANCY D. PERRIER

SURGICAL ONCOLOGY CLINICS OF NORTH AMERICA

www.surgonc.theclinics.com

Consulting Editor
TIMOTHY M. PAWLIK

April 2023 • Volume 32 • Number 2

ELSEVIER

1600 John F. Kennedy Boulevard • Suite 1800 • Philadelphia, Pennsylvania, 19103-2899

http://www.theclinics.com

SURGICAL ONCOLOGY CLINICS OF NORTH AMERICA Volume 32, Number 2
April 2023 ISSN 1055-3207, ISBN-13: 978-0-323-93977-5

Editor: John Vassallo (j.vassallo@elsevier.com)
Developmental Editor: Diana Ang

Surgical Oncology Clinics of North America (ISSN 1055-3207) is published quarterly by Elsevier Inc., 360 Park Avenue South, New York, NY 10010-1710. Months of publication are January, April, July, and October. Business and Editorial Offices: 1600 John F. Kennedy Blvd., Ste. 1800, Philadelphia, PA 19103-2899. Customer Service Office: 3251 Riverport Lane, Maryland Heights, MO 63043. Periodicals postage paid at New York, NY and additional mailing offices. Subscription prices are $335.00 per year (US individuals), $651.00 (US institutions) $100.00 (US student/resident), $374.00 (Canadian individuals), $823.00 (Canadian institutions), $100.00 (Canadian student/resident), $484.00 (foreign individuals), $823.00 (foreign institutions), and $205.00 (foreign student/resident). Foreign air speed delivery is included in all *Clinics* subscription prices. All prices are subject to change without notice. **POSTMASTER**: Send address changes to *Surgical Oncology Clinics of North America,* Elsevier Health Science Division, Subscription Customer Service, 3251 Riverport Lane, Maryland Heights, MO 63043. **Customer Service: 1-800-654-2452 (US and Canada). 314-447-8871 (outside US and Canada). Fax: 314-447-8029. E-mail: journalscustomerservice-usa@elsevier.com (for print support); journalsonline support-usa@elsevier.com (for online support)**.

Reprints. For copies of 100 or more, of articles in this publication, please contact the Commercial Reprints Department, Elsevier Inc., 360 Park Avenue South, New York, New York 10010-1710. Tel. 212-633-3874; Fax: 212-633-3820; E-mail: reprints@elsevier.com.

Surgical Oncology Clinics of North America is covered in *MEDLINE/PubMed (Index Medicus) and EMBASE/ Excerpta Medica, Current Contents/Clinical Medicine, and ISI/BIOMED.*

Contributors

CONSULTING EDITOR

TIMOTHY M. PAWLIK, MD, PhD, MPH, MTS, MBA, FACS, FSSO, FRACS (Hon.)
Professor and Chair, Department of Surgery, The Urban Meyer III and Shelley Meyer Chair for Cancer Research, Professor of Surgery, Oncology, Health Services Management and Policy, The Ohio State University, Wexner Medical Center, Columbus, Ohio, USA

EDITOR

NANCY D. PERRIER, MD, FACS
Ruth and Walter Sterling Endowed Professor of Surgery, Chief, Surgical Endocrinology, Department of Surgical Oncology, The University of Texas MD Anderson Cancer Center, Houston, Texas, USA

AUTHORS

MARIA F. BATES, MD, FACS
Assistant Professor of Surgery, Geisel School of Medicine at Dartmouth, Hanover, New Hampshire, USA; Endocrine Surgeon, Department of Surgery, Dartmouth-Hitchcock Medical Center, Section of General Surgery, Lebanon, New Hampshire, USA

THOMAS C. BECK, PhD
Department of Surgery, Stanford University, School of Medicine, Stanford, California, USA

LODEWIJK A.A. BROSENS, MD, PhD
Department of Pathology, University Medical Center Utrecht, Utrecht, the Netherlands

URIEL CLEMENTE-GUTIERREZ, MD
Department of Surgical Oncology, Division of Surgical Endocrinology, The University of Texas MD Anderson Cancer Center, Houston, Texas, USA

SETH J. CONCORS, MD
Complex General Surgical Oncology Fellow, Department of Surgical Oncology, The University of Texas MD Anderson Cancer Center, Houston, Texas, USA

OLIVER J. FACKELMAYER, MD
Division of General, Endocrine and Metabolic Surgery, Assistant Professor of Surgery, General, Endocrine and Metabolic Surgery, University of Kentucky, Lexington, Kentucky, USA

MARYBETH HUGHES, MD, FACS
Professor, Department of Surgery, Chief, Division of Surgical Oncology, Eastern Virginia Medical School, Norfolk, Virginia, USA

NARUHIKO IKOMA, MD, MS
Assistant Professor and Director of Minimally-Invasive Surgical Oncology Program, Department of Surgical Oncology, The University of Texas MD Anderson Cancer Center, Houston, Texas, USA

WILLIAM B. INABNET III, MD, MHA, FACS
Division of General, Endocrine and Metabolic Surgery, University of Kentucky, Johnston-Wright Endowed Professor and Chair, Department of Surgery, University of Kentucky College of Medicine, Surgeon-in-Chief, UK HealthCare, Lexington, Kentucky, USA

ISABELLA MARÉCHAL-ROSS, MD
Endocrine Surgery Unit, Royal North Shore Hospital, Northern Sydney Local Health District and Northern Clinical School, Sydney Medical School, Faculty of Medicine and Health, University of Sydney, St Leonards, New South Wales, Australia

MATTHEW H.G. KATZ, MD
Professor and Chair, Department of Surgical Oncology, The University of Texas MD Anderson Cancer Center, Houston, Texas, USA

ELECTRON KEBEBEW, MD
Department of Surgery, Stanford University, School of Medicine, Stanford, California, USA

LISA KENNEY, MD
Resident Physician, Department of Surgery, Eastern Virginia Medical School, Norfolk, Virginia, USA

MICHAEL S. LUI, MD
Department of Surgical Oncology, Division of Surgical Endocrinology, The University of Texas MD Anderson Cancer Center, Houston, Texas, USA

ROBERT MECHERA, MD, Dr med habil
Endocrine Surgery Unit, Royal North Shore Hospital, Northern Sydney Local Health District and Northern Clinical School, Sydney Medical School, Faculty of Medicine and Health, University of Sydney, St Leonards, New South Wales, Australia; Clarunis, University Hospital Basel, Basel, Switzerland; Endocrine and Breast Surgery, St. George Hospital, Kogarah, New South Wales, Australia

RADU MIHAI, MD, PhD, FRCS
Consultant Endocrine Surgeon, Endocrine Surgery Unit, Churchill Cancer Centre, Oxford University Hospitals NHS Foundation Trust, Oxford, United Kingdom

NARIS NILUBOL, MD, FACS
Surgical Oncology Program, Endocrine Surgery Section, National Cancer Institute, National Institutes of Health, Bethesda, Maryland, USA

NANCY D. PERRIER, MD, FACS
Ruth and Walter Sterling Endowed Professor of Surgery, Chief, Surgical Endocrinology, Department of Surgical Oncology, The University of Texas MD Anderson Cancer Center, Houston, Texas, USA

PETER CAMPBELL, MBBS, FRACS
Sydney Medical School, Faculty of Medicine and Health, University of Sydney, Sydney, New South Wales, Australia

CAROLINA R.C. PIETERMAN, MD, PhD
Department of Endocrine Oncology, University Medical Center, Utrecht, the Netherlands

BHAVISHYA RAMAMOORTHY, MD
Surgical Oncology Program, Endocrine Surgery Section, National Cancer Institute, National Institutes of Health, Bethesda, Maryland, USA

CAROLYN D. SEIB, MD, MAS
Department of Surgery, Stanford–Surgery Policy Improvement Research and Education Center (S-SPIRE), Stanford University School of Medicine, Stanford, California, USA

STAN B. SIDHU, PhD, FRACS
Endocrine Surgery Unit, Royal North Shore Hospital, Northern Sydney Local Health District and Northern Clinical School, Sydney Medical School, Faculty of Medicine and Health, University of Sydney, St Leonards, New South Wales, Australia

ANGELICA M. SILVA-FIGUEROA, MD, MEd, FACS
Universidad Finis Terrae, School of Medicine, Chile; Service of Surgery, Department of Head and Neck Surgery, Hospital Barros Luco Trudeau, Santiago, Chile

CATHERINE M. SKEFOS, MA, MS
Clinical Cancer Genetics Program, Division of Surgical Endocrinology, The University of Texas MD Anderson Cancer Center, Houston, Texas, USA

MEREDITH J. SORENSEN, MD, MS, FACS
Assistant Professor of Surgery, Geisel School of Medicine at Dartmouth, Hanover, New Hampshire, USA; Section of General Surgery, Division Chief of Endocrine Surgery, Department of Surgery, Dartmouth-Hitchcock Medical Center, Lebanon, New Hampshire, USA

MARK S. SYWAK, MMed, FRACS
Endocrine Surgery Unit, Royal North Shore Hospital, Northern Sydney Local Health District and Northern Clinical School, Sydney Medical School, Faculty of Medicine and Health, University of Sydney, St Leonards, New South Wales, Australia; Endocrine and Breast Surgery, St. George Hospital, Kogarah, New South Wales, Australia

MAY THWIN, MBBS, MClinSci, FRACS
Fellow in Endocrine Surgery, Endocrine Surgery Unit, Churchill Cancer Centre, Oxford University Hospitals NHS Foundation Trust, Oxford, United Kingdom

GERLOF D. VALK, MD, PhD
Department of Endocrine Oncology, University Medical Center, Utrecht, the Netherlands

DIRK-JAN VAN BEEK, MD, PhD, MSc
Department of Endocrine Surgical Oncology, University Medical Center Utrecht, Utrecht, the Netherlands

ANNA VERA D. VERSCHUUR, MD
Department of Pathology, University Medical Center Utrecht, Utrecht, the Netherlands

MENNO R. VRIENS, MD, PhD
Department of Endocrine Surgical Oncology, University Medical Center Utrecht, Utrecht, the Netherlands

Contents

Foreword: Surgical Endocrinology xiii

Timothy M. Pawlik

Preface: Special Edition on Surgical Endocrinology in Honor of Orlo H. Clark xv

Nancy D. Perrier

A Contemporary Review of the Treatment of Medullary Thyroid Carcinoma in the Era of New Drug Therapies 233

Carolyn D. Seib, Thomas C. Beck, and Electron Kebebew

Medullary thyroid cancer (MTC) is a rare neuroendocrine tumor that can be sporadic or inherited and is often associated with mutations in the RET (Rearranged during Transfection) oncogene. The primary treatment for MTC is surgical resection of all suspected disease, but recent advances in targeted therapies for MTC, including the selective RET inhibitors selpercatinib and pralsetinib, have led to changes in the management of patients with locally advanced, metastatic, or recurrent MTC. In this article, we review updates on the evaluation and management of patients with MTC, focusing on new and emerging therapies that are likely to improve patient outcomes.

A Nomogram for Relapse/Death and Contemplating Adjuvant Therapy for Parathyroid Carcinoma 251

Angelica M. Silva-Figueroa

Parathyroid carcinoma (PC) is a rare endocrine malignancy with an increased incidence in the last decade. There is no reliable prognostic staging system for PC. Several hosts, tumors, and tumor microenvironment factors have been negatively correlated with survival in the last decade. Surgical resection with negative margins is still the standard of treatment in PC. Chemo and radiotherapy have no proven beneficial effect. A new promising approach with molecular profiling could lead to adjuvant therapies.

Parathyroid Cancer: Updates and Postoperative Surveillance Imaging 271

May Thwin and Radu Mihai

Imaging after definitive surgical management of parathyroid carcinoma remains a poorly defined area, and at present, there are no standard guidelines to direct care, which should be individualized and patient-oriented. The current role of imaging is largely reserved for patients who demonstrate biochemical or clinical evidence to suggest disease recurrence, and in these patients, imaging is directed at identifying the culprit site of disease to direct further surgery. There is no established role for “routine” or “surveillance” imaging in those patients with sporadic who do not display signs of disease recurrence.

Adjuvant and neoadjuvant chemotherapy in the treatment of adrenocortical carcinoma (ACC) is limited by few existing trials, most of which are retrospective. The drug mitotane has been used for the treatment of ACC, although existing guidelines only support its use in high risk of recurrence. The first phase 3 trial involving systemic chemotherapy for ACC supports the use of etoposide, doxorubicin, cisplatin, and mitotane for combination therapy. No significant breakthrough has been discovered thus far in of targeted and immunotherapies. Neoadjuvant chemotherapy is only used to allow for complete surgical resection because complete excision is the definitive treatment of ACC.

It is recognized that a large portion of pheochromocytoma and paraganglioma cases will have an underlying germline mutation, supporting the recommendation for universal genetic testing in all patients with PPGLs. A mutation in succinate dehydrogenase subunit B is associated with increased rates of developing synchronous and/or metachronous metastatic disease. Patients identified with this mutation require meticulous preoperative evaluation, a personalized surgical plan to minimize the risk of recurrence and tumor spread, and lifelong surveillance.

Surgical diseases of the adrenal gland include pheochromocytoma/paraganglioma, primary hyperaldosteronism, Cushing syndrome, and adrenocortical carcinoma. These conditions may be associated with familial syndromes, and genetic testing is available and recommended in most. Adrenal surgeons should be familiar with these syndromes and know when to consider referral for genetic counseling and genetic testing. Identification of patients with familial syndromes allows for the detection and screening of associated syndromic neoplasms, guides surgical planning and operative approach, influences recurrence and malignancy risk assessment, aids in the development of a postoperative surveillance plan, and determines the need for screening family members.

Multiple endocrine neoplasia type 1 syndrome (MEN1) is a disease caused by mutations in the MEN1 tumor suppressor gene leading to hyperparathyroidism, pituitary adenomas, and entero-pancreatic neuroendocrine tumors. Pancreatic neuroendocrine tumors (PNETs) are a major cause of mortality in patients with MEN1. Identification of consistent genotype–phenotype correlations has remained elusive, but MEN1 mutations in exons 2, 9, and 10 may be associated with metastatic PNETs; patients with these mutations may benefit from more intensive surveillance and aggressive treatment. In addition, epigenetic differences between MEN1-associated PNETs and sporadic PNETs are beginning to emerge, but further investigation is required to establish clear phenotypic associations.

Minimally invasive pancreatectomy is increasingly used. Although offering potential advantages over open approaches, minimally invasive pancreatectomy has many challenges to maintain high-quality of oncologic resection. Multiple patient and surgical factors should be considered in planning laparoscopic or robotic resection, including the learning curve required to produce proficiency. For pancreaticoduodenectomy, distal pancreatectomy, and other pancreatic resections, a safe, margin-negative resection remains the goal. National and societal guidelines for the adoption of minimally invasive pancreatectomy are ongoing and will continue to be important as these techniques are further adopted.

Pancreatic neuroendocrine tumors (PNETs) occur in < 1/100,000 patients and most are nonfunctioning (NF). Approximately 5% occur as part of multiple endocrine neoplasia type 1. Anatomic and molecular imaging have a pivotal role in the diagnosis, staging and active surveillance. Surgery is generally recommended for nonfunctional pancreatic neuroendocrine tumors (NF-PNETs) >2 cm to prevent metastases. For tumors ≤2 cm, active surveillance is a viable alternative. Tumor size and grade are important factors to guide management. Assessment of death domain-associated protein 6/alpha-thalassemia/mental retardation X-linked and alternative lengthening of telomeres are promising novel prognostic markers. This review summarizes the status of surveillance and nonsurgical management for small NF-PNETs, including factors that can guide management.

Thyroid surgery remains an essential treatment of thyroid cancer. The historical one-size-fits-all approach to differentiated (papillary and follicular) thyroid carcinoma of total thyroidectomy with central lymph node dissection has been shown to be overtreatment with associated risk of perioperative complications including nerve palsy and hypoparathyroidism. Furthermore, thyroid lobectomy may obviate life-long thyroid hormone replacement. Low-risk thyroid cancers have a low risk of recurrence and those that do recur can be salvaged with reoperation without compromising prognosis. Perioperative risk stratification for recurrence and death greatly influence the need for total thyroidectomy.

Lymph node metastasis in thyroid cancer is common and associated with an increased risk of locoregional recurrence (LRR). Although therapeutic central neck dissection is well established, prophylactic central node dissection (pCND) for microscopic occult nodal involvement is controversial and recommendations are based on low-level evidence. The potential benefits of pCND such as reducing LRR and re-operation, refining staging, and improving surveillance are enthusiastically debated and the decision to perform pCND must be weighed up against the increased risks of complications.

SURGICAL ONCOLOGY CLINICS OF NORTH AMERICA

SERIES OF RELATED INTEREST

Advances in Surgery
https://www.advancessurgery.com
Surgical Clinics of North America
https://www.surgical.theclinics.com
Thoracic Surgery Clinics
https://www.thoracic.theclinics.com

THE CLINICS ARE AVAILABLE ONLINE!
Access your subscription at:
www.theclinics.com

Foreword

Surgical Endocrinology

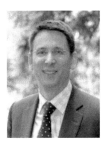

Timothy M. Pawlik,
MD, PhD, MPH,
MTS, MBA, FACS,
FSSO, FRACS (Hon.)
Consulting Editor

This issue of the *Surgical Oncology Clinics of North America* focuses on surgical endocrinology. Surgery of the thyroid, parathyroid, adrenal, and endocrine pancreas has been performed for centuries as part of general surgery. Only in the twentieth century did surgeons begin to consider the endocrine system in a more holistic way, incorporating an understanding of underlying hormonal/chemical perturbations with anatomic organs. During the twentieth century, there were many surgical pioneers in endocrine surgery that addressed newly defined diseases and syndromes. For example, Sir John Bland Sutton performed the first parathyroidectomy in London around 1918, while adrenalectomy for pheochromocytoma was performed by Cesar Roux in Lausanne and by Charles Mayo in 1926. Other pioneers included Theodor Kocher, Thomas Dunhill, and George Crile, who pioneered safe thyroid surgery. In the early 1970s, the world's first-ever course on endocrine surgery was established at the Hammersmith Hospital.[1] This course brought together the world's leaders in the field and established Hammersmith Hospital as a center of endocrine surgery. From 1970 to 1971, Dr Orlo Clark was an endocrine surgical fellow with Mr Selwyn Taylor and Professor Richard Welbourn at Hammersmith Hospital. Later, Dr Clark would note that the timing was right for the development of endocrine surgery as a specialty outside of general surgery.[1] Dr Clark, in conjunction with Drs Norman Thompson, Edwin Kaplan, Jack Monchik, and Tony Edis, would go on to start the American Association of Endocrine Surgeons. With the recent passing of Dr Clark, it is only appropriate that we dedicate this issue of *Surgical Oncology Clinics of North America* to Dr Clark and his profound scientific and clinical impact on surgical endocrinology. In turn, I am grateful to have Nancy D. Perrier, MD, FACS as the guest editor of this important issue of *Surgical Oncology Clinics of North America*. Dr Perrier is the Ruth and Walter Sterling Endowed Professor of Surgery, as well as Chief of Surgical Endocrinology at The University of Texas MD Anderson Cancer

Surg Oncol Clin N Am 32 (2023) xiii–xiv
https://doi.org/10.1016/j.soc.2023.01.001
1055-3207/23/© 2023 Published by Elsevier Inc.

surgonc.theclinics.com

Center. Dr Perrier has had a life-long career interest in endocrine neoplasms. Her scholarly works include more than 350 publications, and 42 book chapters. She has extensive experience and leadership in the area of surgical endocrinology and is therefore imminently qualified to be the guest editor of this important issue of *Surgical Oncology Clinics of North America*.

The issue covers a range of important topics related to surgical endocrinology. In particular, the issue highlights contemporary treatment of medullary thyroid carcinoma, postoperative surveillance, and adjuvant therapy for parathyroid carcinoma, as well as multimodality treatment of adrenal tumors, including adrenocortical carcinoma and pheochromocytomas. In addition to these important topics, the authors also provide a contemporary state-of-the-art update on clinical management of pancreatic neuroendocrine tumors. The team of expert coauthors also provide insights into the role of lobectomy versus total thyroidectomy for differentiated thyroid cancer, as well as the role of central neck dissection in the management of such diseases as papillary thyroid carcinoma.

I wish to express my sincere gratitude to Dr Perrier for her efforts to amass such a wonderful group of leaders in the field of surgical endocrinology. These expert authors have done a masterful job outlining the latest updates in surgical endocrinology that will benefit both trainees and faculty. I know that this issue of *Surgical Oncology Clinics of North America* will serve to inform surgeons about the latest up-to-date data on the surgical management of endocrine tumors. Once again, my sincere gratitude to Dr Perrier and all the authors for contributing to this issue of the *Surgical Oncology Clinics of North America*. In addition, we collectively salute the legacy of Dr Orlo Clark for blazing the trail in surgical endocrinology that has benefited so many surgeons, endocrinologists, trainees, and—most importantly—patients.

Timothy M. Pawlik, MD, PhD, MPH, MTS, MBA, FACS, FSSO, FRACS (Hon.)
Professor and Chair
Department of Surgery
The Urban Meyer III and Shelley Meyer Chair for Cancer Research
The Ohio State University
Wexner Medical Center
395 West 12th Avenue, Suite 670
Columbus, OH 43210, USA

E-mail address:
tim.pawlik@osumc.edu

REFERENCE

1. Available at: https://endocrinesurgery.uk/the-history-of-endocrine-surgery/. Accessed December 17, 2022.

Preface

Special Edition on Surgical Endocrinology in Honor of Orlo H. Clark

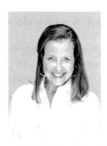

Nancy D. Perrier, MD, FACS
Editor

The history of the specialty of endocrine surgery can be traced back to a group of individuals who shared camaraderie, expertise, passion, and friendship. Among them was Orlo H. Clark, whose memory we honor with this issue. From these roots, an entire family tree of learning has grown that has sprouted into every crevice of the surgical world. Orlo was a class act, pushing those in the specialty to reach our best potential, challenge the status quo, think outside the box, and be inclusive in terms of every aspect of diversity. His photographic memory and brilliance at understanding the scientific literature challenged and inspired multiple generations of surgeons. From the beginning of his career, before we knew the phrase *diversity, equity, and inclusion*, he was a San Francisco giant—both in surgery and in modeling the way. He and his wife Carol traveled extensively as he planted seeds of knowledge, revealing his passion for Asia and his love of Europe and Scandinavia. His curiosity for different cultures and for people was what truly made him stand head and shoulders above everyone in the room. But he always stood slightly bending down, meeting those below him, reaching down to connect with them, acknowledging each person as an individual and being present with them.

This issue is dedicated to Orlo's profound scientific impact on the "little glands" that have output of much importance. This issue brings together young experts from across the globe, authors who are fruits of the vine that Orlo helped established. The topics are those for which he felt such passion: benign and malignant parathyroid disease; principles of thyroid cancer and the role of lymph node dissection, advancing knowledge of MEN1, and improving management and surveillance; teaching the clinical importance of recognizing genetic implications; being aware of rapid advances in medullary thyroid cancer; and spreading excitement about the science of the development and function of pheochromocytoma. These are ideas he would think are worth sharing.

Surg Oncol Clin N Am 32 (2023) xv–xvii
https://doi.org/10.1016/j.soc.2022.10.001
1055-3207/23/© 2022 Published by Elsevier Inc.

surgonc.theclinics.com

The idea of specializing in endocrine surgery began in a liminal space—a thin plane between general, vascular, hepatobiliary, urologic, and head and neck surgery; internal medicine; and endocrinology. Endocrine surgery was initiated on the fringe, not at the center of a defined group of surgeons at that time. This origin was beneficial because when we are at the center of something, we can easily confuse essentials with nonessentials and get tied down by trivial markers of success, loyalty tests, and job security. Not much truth and growth can happen there. Endocrine surgery was on the edge. Orlo recognized that this was an auspicious and advantageous position. He and a few friends had a vision, and he believed in it and the promise that it held for something that would endure. Orlo lived by displaying that the best criticism of the bad is the practice of the better. The idea that the friendly surgeons were endocrine surgeons embodied that genuineness of his demeanor.

In endocrine surgery, trainees learned to risk leaving their own secure systems of training, where surgeons performed operations as pure technicians, and instead pursue true mastery of technical excellence. Orlo encouraged his professional children to leave their home base of surgery and connect with other disciplines, like endocrinology, genetics, pathology, nuclear medicine, oncology, pharmacology, radiology, anesthesia, and basic science. He modeled how to always be hospitable—even amid the hostility of others. His true idea of the endocrine surgery specialty was a world that existed as a place of entrance and exit where people came and went freely, not a place of settlement. He used the specialty to open doors, build bridges, and especially to welcome travelers passing through. Orlo was not an insider throwing rocks at outsiders with the nuances and subtleties of specialization, nor was he comfortable defending the status quo. Instead, he exemplified living precariously with two perspectives holding people together. He was not ensconced safely inside the specialty, where perspective and curiosity are lost, nor situated so far outside as to lose compassion, voice, or understanding. Orlo challenged with a necessary, creative tension and curiosity. It was his true gift and unique kind of seeing and living that created a specialty that offers a lasting invitation to continue engaging with the much larger world embellished with beauty and music and art.

From his legacy as a mentor, teacher, friend, husband, father, scientist, and surgeon, we are able to harvest the wisdom of the cycle of life and science. Experiencing first-hand joys, sorrows, glories, and illuminations—each is necessary, he helped us understand, for the development of an endocrine surgeon and, indeed, a full human being.

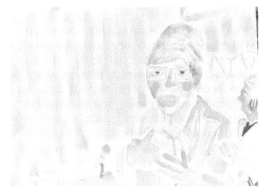

Fig. 1. Orlo at the microphone, recognized by his all stature and long fingers.

Always the teacher, still teaching us now. We could always count on Orlo to come to the microphone and make a thoughtful contribution (**Fig. 1**). Never political, never anything but kind. The relationships he built with every single trainee and fellow were an embodiment of what it means to be inclusive, to open your home and your heart, and to do it with dignity, always thinking of others and doing so with peace and grace.

Nancy D. Perrier, MD, FACS
Surgical Endocrinology, Department of Surgical Oncology, MD Anderson Cancer Center, Houston, TX, USA

E-mail address:
Nperrier@mdanderson.org

FURTHER READINGS

Cheah WK, Arici C, Ituarte PH, al eta. Complications of neck dissection for thyroid cancer. World J Surg 2002;26(8):1013–6.

Clark OH. Thyroid cancer and lymph node metastases. J Surg Oncol 2011;103(6):615–8.

Fernandez-Ranvier GG, Khanafshar E, Jensen K, et al. Parathyroid carcinoma, atypical parathyroid adenoma or parathyromatosis? Cancer 2007;110(2):255–64.

Guerrero MA, Lindsay S, Suh I, et al. Medullary thyroid cancer: it is a pain in the neck? J Cancer 2011;2:200–5.

Zarnegar R, Brunaud L, Clark OH. Multiple endocrine neoplasia type 1. Curr Treat Options Oncol 2002;3(4):335–48.

Zarnegar R, Kebebew E, Duh QY, et al. Malignant pheochromocytoma. Surg Oncol Clin N Am 2006;15(3):555–71.

A Contemporary Review of the Treatment of Medullary Thyroid Carcinoma in the Era of New Drug Therapies

Carolyn D. Seib, MD, MAS[a,b], Thomas C. Beck, PhD[b],
Electron Kebebew, MD[b],*

KEYWORDS

- Medullary thyroid carcinoma • Neuroendocrine tumor • Thyroidectomy
- Lymph node dissection • Targeted therapy • Medullary thyroid cancer • *RET*

KEY POINTS

- Medullary thyroid cancer (MTC) can be sporadic or inherited in patients with multiple endocrine neoplasia type 2 (MEN2): MEN2A and MEN2B.
- Screening and surveillance for MTC and prophylactic thyroidectomy is associated with improved outcomes in patients with germline *RET* proto-oncogene mutations.
- Preoperative calcitonin and carcinoembryonic antigen (CEA) levels can guide meticulous surgical resection of all suspected diseases at initial MTC diagnosis and guide initial imaging studies that are necessary for appropriate staging.
- Fluorine-18-l-dihydroxyphenylalanine or [68]gallium DOTATATE imaging can be useful in patients with recurrent or persistent disease.
- The selective RET (Rearranged during Transfection) inhibitors selpercatinib and pralsetinib have been approved for the management of patients with progressive locally advanced or metastatic MTC and hold promise to greatly improve outcomes.

INTRODUCTION

Medullary thyroid cancer (MTC) is a neuroendocrine tumor derived from parafollicular cells (C cells) that accounts for 1% to 2% of thyroid cancer cases.[1] MTC can be sporadic or inherited. Hereditary MTC accounts for approximately 25% of all MTC cases and is referred to as multiple endocrine neoplasia type 2 (MEN2): MEN2A, MEN2B,

[a] Surgery Policy Improvement Research and Education Center (S-SPIRE), Stanford University School of Medicine, 300 Pasteur Drive H3642, Stanford, CA 94305, USA; [b] Department of Surgery, Stanford University, School of Medicine, 300 Pasteur Drive H3642, Stanford, CA 94305, USA
* Corresponding author.
E-mail address: kebebew@stanford.edu

Surg Oncol Clin N Am 32 (2023) 233–250
https://doi.org/10.1016/j.soc.2022.10.002
1055-3207/23/© 2022 Elsevier Inc. All rights reserved.

surgonc.theclinics.com

and familial MTC (now defined as a subtype of MEN2A) (**Table 1**). Germline mutations in the *RET* (Rearranged during Transfection) oncogene are present in almost all patients with inherited forms of MTC. Somatic mutations in *RET* are present in approximately 66% of sporadic cases, and somatic *RAS* mutations are also common.[2] The mainstay of treatment of MTC is meticulous surgical resection of all suspected diseases at initial diagnosis. Unlike differentiated thyroid cancers, MTC is not susceptible to radioactive iodine treatment. As a result, the management of persistent and recurrent MTC was historically addressed with reoperation or radiation therapy with variable success and significant associated morbidity. To address this clinical challenge, recent advances in targeted therapies for MTC have led to changes in standard treatment protocols in the setting of advanced-stage disease and improved long-term outcomes for patients with locally advanced, metastatic, or recurrent MTC. This article reviews updates on the pathobiology, evaluation, prognosis, and treatment of patients with MTC in the era of new and targeted therapies, in addition to treatments under investigation that may further improve the management of patients with this neuroendocrine tumor.

PATHOBIOLOGY OF MEDULLARY THYROID CANCER

Activating point mutations in *RET* and *RAS* result in MTC. The nature of *RET* mutation (germline vs somatic), location, and variant inform the treatment and prognosis of MTC. The most common genetic mutations associated with sporadic MTCs are in the *RET* and *RAS* oncogenes. Approximately 50% of sporadic MTCs are caused by mutations in *RET*. Approximately 40% of RET mutation-negative sporadic MTC is caused by mutations in *RAS*. On the contrary, germline *RET* mutations are responsible for nearly all cases of inherited MTCs that are associated with the development of MEN2A and MEN2B syndromes. [3,4]

RET is a proto-oncogene that is located on the long arm of chromosome 10 (10q11.2). It encodes for a transmembrane receptor tyrosine kinase expressed in mostly organs that derive from the embryologic neural crest, including parafollicular C cells in the thyroid gland. The RET receptor is composed of three different domains: an N-terminal extracellular domain, a transmembrane cysteine-rich region, and a cytoplasmic domain with kinase activity. RET kinase is stimulated by tripartite complex formation with glial cell line-derived neurotrophic growth factor (GDNF) family ligands binding to glycosylphosphatidylinositol-linked co-receptor.[5] Stimulation of RET kinase results in downstream signaling of mitogen activated protein kinase (MAPK), phosphatidylinositol 3-kinases (PI3K), and protein kinase B, focal adhesion kinase, signal transducer and activator of transcription (STAT), and steroid receptor coactivator-1 (Src1) pathways that lead to cell survival, differentiation, migration, and proliferation. Disruption of the integrity of this tripartite complex, as well as the structure and function of the RET receptor, can drive the development of disease. For example, mutations in *RET* result in loss or gain of function mutations in the RET kinase signaling pathway. Loss of function mutations is associated with Hirschsprung disease.[6] Gain of function mutations in *RET* is linked with malignancies, such as breast, prostate, pancreatic, myeloid, and thyroid cancers.[5]

Activating point mutations of *RET* are commonly associated with inherited and sporadic MTC.[7] This is in contrast with papillary thyroid carcinoma, which is associated with chromosomal rearrangements that affect RET kinase function.[8] MEN2A is associated with activating point mutations in the *RET* cysteine codons 609, 610, 611, 618, and 620 in exon 10 and Cys634Arg in exon 11. These mutations lead to the ligand-independent constitutive activation of RET kinase signaling via disulfide-bonded homodimers. MEN2B is associated with Met918Thr in exon 16 of *RET* that leads to

Table 1
Classification and clinical manifestations of inherited medullary thyroid cancer

	Subtype	Clinical Manifestations
MEN2A	Classical	Medullary thyroid cancer, pheochromocytoma, and primary hyperparathyroidism
	Subtypes with additional clinical features	w/Cutaneous lichen amyloidosis
		w/Hirschsprung disease[a]
		Familial MTC
MEN2B		Medullary thyroid cancer, pheochromocytoma, mucosal neuromas, intestinal ganglioneuromas, and marfanoid habitus

Abbreviation: MTC, medullary thyroid cancer.

[a] *RET* mutations in exon 10, especially affecting codons 618 and 620.

constitutive activation via promoting a high level of autophosphorylation of RET receptors. Interestingly, there is geographic variability between the *RET* variants that are linked with the development of MEN2A.[9] Specific germline *RET* variants are correlated with age of presentation and aggressiveness of MTC, and the occurrence of other manifestation (pheochromocytoma, primary hyperparathyroidism), and this genotype-phenotype association has been used to determine the optimal age for the initiation of screening and surveillance, as well as recommending early total thyroidectomy (**Table 2**).[10–12] Screening and surveillance for MTC in patients with germline *RET* mutations is associated with the improved outcome due to early detection of MTC or before MTC develops.[10,11,13–15] The most frequent somatic mutation associated with sporadic MTC is Met918Thr, which is commonly found in MEN2B.[8] Among sporadic MTC, a proportion of *RET* mutation-negative tumors (approximately 40%) are associated with mutations in *RAS*, a downstream signaling molecule of RET signaling.[4,16] An even smaller proportion of MTC has genetic causes of unknown origin.

DIAGNOSIS AND OPTIMAL IMAGING STRATEGY

Medullary thyroid cancer is most commonly diagnosed based on cytology from fine-needle aspiration (FNA) biopsy in a patient with one or more thyroid nodules. The FNA biopsy has a reported sensitivity of 89% (range 63% to 94%) for MTC.[17] In addition to cytologic features characteristic of MTC, including plasmacytoid or spindled cells, dyshesion, multinucleation, salt-and-pepper chromatin, and the presence of amyloid, calcitonin immunostaining is performed to confirm the diagnosis.[18] Clinicians should be aware that MTC, depending on subtype, can mimic follicular or Hürthle cell neoplasms, and immunostaining with calcitonin, CEA, and thyroglobulin may be necessary when there is diagnostic uncertainty.[17] Guidelines leave it to the clinician's discretion whether to perform routine measurement of serum calcitonin in patients presenting with nodular thyroid disease.[1] A 2020 Cochrane review analyzed 16 studies, accounting for over 70,000 patients with nodular thyroid disease who had routine calcitonin testing, and found serum calcitonin to have a higher median sensitivity and specificity for MTC (99.7% and 99.6%, respectively) than typically reported for FNA, but a low positive predictive value (PPV) of 7.7% given the low prevalence of disease (0.32% median prevalence of MTC in this population).[19] Given this low PPV and the potential for study bias due to incomplete follow-up of patients with negative calcitonin screening, the authors concluded that the value of routine testing of calcitonin in nodular thyroid disease remains questionable, which is consistent with published guidelines.

Initial evaluation after diagnosis of MTC includes cervical ultrasound with lymph node mapping and FNA of any lateral compartment lymph nodes suspicious for metastatic disease. Ultrasound is more sensitive and specific than computed tomography (CT) scan for identifying MTC and associated lymphadenopathy, and both the American Thyroid Association (ATA) sonographic risk patterns and the thyroid imaging reporting and data system (TI-RADS) criteria perform well in classifying MTC nodules as high risk (**Fig. 1**).[20–22] In addition, patients should undergo evaluation of tumor markers (eg, calcitonin and CEA) and genetic testing for germline *RET* mutations. Before surgical resection, plasma fractionated metanephrines and/or 24-h urine metanephrines and serum calcium and parathyroid hormone (PTH) should be measured to evaluate for conditions associated with MEN2, pheochromocytoma and primary hyperparathyroidism, respectively. If a pheochromocytoma is diagnosed, this should be addressed with alpha blockade and adrenalectomy first, with prompt management of MTC subsequently. If primary hyperparathyroidism is identified, concurrent parathyroidectomy should be performed during thyroidectomy for MTC and it is usually due to single parathyroid gland disease.

If the serum calcitonin concentration is greater than 500 pg/mL or in patients with extensive neck disease, the initial workup should also include evaluation for distant metastases with contrast-enhanced CT scans of the neck, chest, abdomen, and pelvis.[1] Liver metastases in MTC can be very small or miliary and are best identified with dynamic, contrast-enhanced liver MRI followed by multiphase abdomen CT with non-enhanced, late arterial phase, portal venous phase, and delayed phase imaging.[23,24] In patients with significantly elevated calcitonin levels (>500 to 1000 pg/mL), PET imaging may be helpful to identify locoregional or distant metastases. The best radionuclide for the identification of MTC metastases is fluorine-18-l-dihydroxyphenylalanine (^{18}F-DOPA), which has better sensitivity and specificity than 18F-fluorodeoxyglucose PET.[25–28] The performance of all nuclear medicine imaging studies in detecting metastatic or recurrent MTC improves with increasing calcitonin levels.[29,30] ^{18}F-DOPA or [68]gallium DOTATATE imaging can be useful in patients with calcitonin >500 pg/mL at diagnosis or those with recurrent or persistent disease and calcitonin levels greater than 150 pg/mL (see **Fig. 1**).[31,32]

SURGICAL MANAGEMENT OF MEDULLARY THYROID CANCER

The initial surgical management of biopsy-proven MTC is dependent primarily on the presence of lateral neck lymph node metastases and calcitonin/CEA levels. The recommended treatment of node-negative MTC in adults is total thyroidectomy with bilateral central neck lymph node dissection, due to the high risk of occult central compartment lymph node metastases. In children with small tumors and minimal elevation in serum calcitonin levels, ipsilateral central neck dissection may be appropriate given the increased risk and potential morbidity of hypoparathyroidism in this population. There is no consensus on the role of prophylactic lateral neck dissections based on current published guidelines.[1,33,34] Performance of prophylactic ipsilateral or bilateral lateral neck dissections (without clinical or radiologic evidence of metastatic disease) in patients with high serum levels of tumor markers is supported by observational data showing that the risks of ipsilateral central and lateral and contralateral central and lateral lymph node metastases increase incrementally with increasing serum calcitonin and CEA levels among a cohort of patients with both sporadic and familial MTC.[35] In addition, increasing primary tumor size is associated with an

Table 2
Screening, manifestations, and treatment for patients based on specific *RET* (rearranged during transfection) gene mutations

RET Mutation(s)	Risk for MTC	Recommended Age to Begin MTC Annual Screening	Recommended Age for Early Thyroidectomy	RET Mutation(s)	Risk for Primary Hyperparathyroidism	RET Mutation(s)	Risk for Pheochromocytoma
918	Highest	Not applicable	In the first months of life	631 634	Approximately 30%	631 634 883 918	Approximately 50%
634,883	High	3 years	At or before age 5 years	618 804 891	<10%	609 611 618 620 630	Approximately 30%
533 609 611 618 620 630 666 768 790 804 891 912	Moderate	3 years	Childhood or young adulthood	515 533 609 611 618 620 918 804 852 883	–	533 666 768 790 804 852 883	Approximately 10%

Abbreviation: MTC, medullary thyroid cancer.

Data from Wells SA, Asa SL, Dralle H, et al. Revised American Thyroid Association Guidelines for the Management of Medullary Thyroid Carcinoma. Thyroid. 2015/06/01 2015;25(6):567-610. https://doi.org/10.1089/thy.2014.0335.

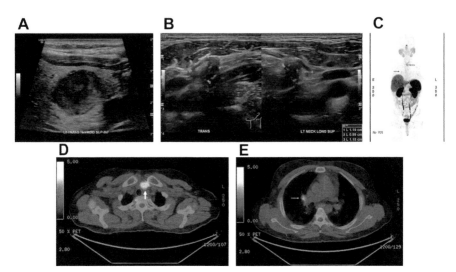

Fig. 1. Imaging features of medullary thyroid cancer on ultrasound and [68]gallium DOTATATE. (*A*) Ultrasound shows a left mid thyroid nodule measuring 1.9 cm with a TI-RADS of 4: Moderately suspicious (composition: solid or almost completely solid [2 points], echogenicity: hypoechoic: hypoechoic compared with adjacent thyroid [2 points], shape: wider-than-tall or width = tall on transverse view [0 points], margin: smooth [0 points]) and (*B*) left abnormal lateral cervical lymph nodes (cervical level 2 [mid]); size: 0.7 cm × 0.4 cm × 0.4 cm, location: lateral to the medial edge of the common carotid artery but medial to the lateral edge of the sternocleidomastoid muscle, (sonographic features: round, Echogenicity: hypoechoic). DOTATATE scan shows (*C*) MIP image showing right lung and mediastinal uptake and fused PET CT showing left mediastinal (*White arrow shows tumor site*) (*D*) and right lung (*White arrow shows tumor site*) (*E*) uptake of [68]gallium DOTATATE (*White arrow shows tumor site*).

increased risk of lymph node metastases,[36] so there should be some consideration for ipsilateral lateral neck dissection in patients with larger primary tumors. However, the risks of lateral neck dissection, including chyle leak and spinal accessory nerve injury, should be carefully weighed when considering an individual patient's risk of occult metastases and incorporated into shared decision-making with individual patients when making decisions about prophylactic lateral neck dissection.[37] Furthermore, a staged approach to the lateral neck compartment after initial total thyroidectomy and bilateral central neck dissection that is guided by the postoperative calcitonin and CEA levels is also an alternative approach.

The penetrance for MTC is nearly 100% in patients with germline *RET* mutations, so prophylactic total thyroidectomy is indicated to prevent or lead to a definitive cure of MTC by intervening before the development of a primary tumor or lymph node metastases (see **Table 2**).[11,15] The timing of prophylactic thyroidectomy is based on the following: (1) the specific *RET* mutation the patient harbors, which dictates the anticipated time to progression from normal C cell to C cell hyperplasia, MTC, locoregional metastases, and distant metastases; and, in some cases; and (2) the serum calcitonin level (basal and/or stimulated). Early central neck dissection should also be performed in children with a preoperative serum calcitonin level greater than 40 pg/mL and those with a codon 918 mutation.[1] Owing to heterogeneity in the timing of disease onset and progression even among established kindred with MEN2, annual surveillance with physical examination, neck ultrasound, and serum calcitonin are warranted starting at age 3. Prophylactic thyroidectomy should be performed by experienced surgeons at tertiary referral centers with expertise in MEN2 to reduce the risk of complications in pediatric patients.[38] It is optimal to delay prophylactic thyroidectomy in those with mutations known to lead to MTC at older ages because of the increased risks and potential adverse effects of hypothyroidism (due to insufficient thyroid hormone replacement during key times for growth and development), hypoparathyroidism, and recurrent laryngeal nerve injury in children.[1]

ADJUVANT THERAPY FOR MEDULLARY THYROID CANCER

The goal of adjuvant radiation therapy in MTC is to prevent or provide local control of disease in patients at high risk of locoregional recurrence. There is data to support external beam radiation therapy (EBRT) to prevent recurrent local disease, but definitive data supporting a benefit to overall survival (OS) are lacking.[39,40] A recent systematic review and meta-analysis including data from 27 nonrandomized studies found that EBRT for MTC with lymph node metastases, microscopic residual disease, or extrathyroidal extension was associated with a 38% reduction in locoregional recurrence but had no association with OS, with data from multiple studies favoring doses of greater than 60 Gy.[41] However, the interpretation of these data is limited based on nonrandom treatment assignment, with patients having higher risk disease being more likely to receive radiation therapy. Morbidity experienced with radiation therapy included dysphagia leading to temporary or permanent enteral feeding (23% and 7%, respectively), short and long-term xerostemia (3% and 7%, respectively), skin desquamation (14%), and fibrosis (20%).[41] Therefore, the potential harms of EBRT in high-risk patients should be weighed against the anticipated benefits related to local control and take into consideration the potential response to systemic targeted therapies (described below).

There is no role for cytotoxic chemotherapy in the management of patients with persistent or recurrent MTC, especially since the advent of tyrosine kinase inhibitor (TKI) therapy. Historical chemotherapy regimens for patients with MTC included therapy with dacarbazine in combination with other agents, including vincristine, cyclophosphamide, sterptozocin, and doxorubicin. However, only a fraction of patients responded and durable control of disease was uncommon.[42,43]

PROGNOSTIC FACTORS FOR MEDULLARY THYROID CANCER

Staging for MTC is according to the American Joint Committee on Cancer (AJCC) pathological tumor, metastasis (pTNM) criteria.[44] This system takes into account tumor size, the presence and location of lymph node metastases, metastatic disease, and extrathyroidal extension to separate patients into stages I–IV (**Table 3**). Although this is the system endorsed by most guidelines,[1] there is evidence that the AJCC tumor size, node and distant metastasis (TNM) staging system does not accurately predict the prognosis of patients with MTC based on poor discrimination of OS among patients with stage I–III disease.[45,46] Most notably, multiple studies have highlighted the importance of number of metastatic lymph nodes to prognosis in MTC and suggested that this information should be included in updated guidelines.[45,47,48] Similar to staging for differentiated thyroid cancer, dynamic risk stratification is supported to update AJCC staging risk estimates and prognosis based on response to therapy in individual patients (Box 1).[49]

Important prognostic features for MTC include age, stage, number of lymph node metastases, calcitonin and CEA levels and doubling time, tumor doubling time, and Ca19.9 positivity and doubling time. Older age has been associated with poor survival of MTC.[13,53] A recent study analyzing outcomes for 1457 with MTC using Surveillance,

Epidemiology, and End Results (SEER) data found that age 65 years and older was independently associated with disease-specific mortality on multivariable Cox proportional hazards regression accounting for stage, surgical intervention, and number of lymph nodes removed (hazard ratio [HR] age 65 to 79 2.91 [95% CI 1.83 to 4.63], HR age $\geq$ 80 6.71 [95% CI 1.83 to 4.63]).[54] Postoperative calcitonin and CEA doubling times have been associated with overall and time to disease recurrence and survival, with doubling times <6 months indicating poor survival, doubling time 6 months to 2 years associated with intermediate risk of poor survival, and doubling time > 2 years deemed low risk.[50,55] Pathologic features indicating adverse outcomes in MTC include mitotic index $\geq$ 5 per 2 mm^2, Ki-67 proliferative index $\geq$ 5%, and tumor necrosis, which may be helpful to inform prognosis in patients with intermediate-risk doubling times.[52] In addition, tumor volume doubling time has been correlated with OS in patients with metastatic disease. In a cohort study of 43 patients with metastatic MTC, patients with an average structural tumor volume doubling time $\leq$ 1 year had a median OS of 11.1 years (95%CI 7.4 to 14.8) compared with a median of 16.5 years (95%CI 10.3 to 22.6) in those with tumor volume doubling time of 1 to 3 years, and 100% OS in those with doubling times $\geq$ 3 years.[56] Ca19.9 is expressed in MTC and detected in the serum of some patients with advanced MTC.[57–59] In a study cohort of 122 patients with MTC (48 with distant metastases, 18.1% with structural persistent disease, and 32.7% with progressive disease at the end of follow-up), Alcenar and associates found that CA19-9 was significantly higher in those who had disease progression and who died from MTC.[51] In a study of 107 patients with advanced MTC, Lorusso and colleagues[60] also reported that there was a significant association between Ca19.9 positivity, and doubling time of < 6 months and < 1 year with mortality but not with disease progression.

TARGETED THERAPY

Targeted therapies for MTC focus on the specific oncogenic pathways involved in its pathogenesis. The management of patients with metastatic or recurrent MTC has been greatly improved with TKIs that inhibit multiple kinases and, most recently, RET specifically. The multikinase inhibitors vandetinib and cabozantinib, which both are nonselective RET inhibitors, were the first targeted systemic therapies approved for the management of progressive or symptomatic MTC, although they have now been largely replaced as first-line treatment by selective RET TKIs. The small molecule vandetinib targets the RET tyrosine-kinase receptor (TKR), in addition to the EGFR and VEGFR pathways, which contribute to tumor angiogenesis, cell proliferation, and cell migration and are commonly overexpressed in advanced MTC.[61] Cabozantinib targets RET, VEGFR, and MET TKRs. In a multicenter phase III randomized, placebo-controlled trial involving 331 patients with advanced MTC, vandetinib showed therapeutic efficacy based on the primary outcome of progression-free survival (PFS, median PFS 19.3 months for placebo vs 30.5 months for vandetinib) and secondary outcomes of objective response rate and biochemical response.[62] In phase III randomized, placebo-controlled EXAM trial for cabozantinib involving 330 patients with unresectable, locally advanced, or metastatic MTC, the estimated median PFS was 4.0 months for placebo versus 11.2 months for cabozantinib.[63] On final analysis of the EXAM results, cabozantinib did not lead to a statistically significant improvement in OS when compared with placebo (median OS 26.6 vs 21.1 months, HR 0.85 [95% CI 0.64 to 1.12]) but subgroup analyses suggested an increased benefit in patients with a somatic *RET* M918 T mutation.[64] Sorafenib, lenvatinib, and sunitinib are other multikinase inhibitors that have been studied in MTC with less impressive

Table 3
Survival based on TNM staging system and other prognostic factors

Variables	5-year Overall Survival	10-year Overall Survival	Median Survival (months)
TNM stage[a] [46]			
I	95%	–	–
II	91%	–	–
III	89%	–	–
IV	68%	–	–
Calcitonin doubling time[50]			
0 to 6 months	25%	8%	–
6 to 24 months	92%	37%	–
>24 months	100%	100%	–
Ca19.9[51]			
≥18.3 U/mL	–	–	230 (SD 106 to 354)
<18.3	–	–	345 (SD 333 to 358)
Pathologic grade[52]—based on having/not having at least one of the following three features:			
• Mitotic index ≥ 5 per 2 mm^2			
• Ki-67 proliferative index ≥ 5%			
• Tumor necrosis			
High grade	66%	47%	–
Low grade	96%	91%	–

[a] Stage I (T1N0M0), stage II (T23N0M0), stage III (T1-3N1aM0), and stage IV (T1-3N1bM0, T4N0-1bM0, and T1-4N0-1bM1).[44]

> **Box 1**
> **Dynamic risk stratification criteria after treatment of MTC**
>
> Dynamic risk stratification following therapy
> - *Excellent response*: Undetectable calcitonin, CEA in the normal range, no structural disease on imaging or physical examination
> - *Biochemical incomplete response*: A detectable calcitonin or elevated CEA with no structural disease on imaging or physical examination
> - *Structural incomplete response*: Persistent or recurrent structural disease on imaging or physical examination

results and notable toxicities but possible applications as salvage therapy for patients with progressive disease and resistance to other TKIs.[65–69]

Although shown to be effective in slowing or stabilizing advanced MTC, the adverse effect profiles of the multikinase inhibitors vandetanib and cabozantinib are poorly tolerated, leading to dose adjustments and drug cessation in a large number of patients in clinical trials and limiting their use in clinical practice.[70] The most common side effects include nausea, fatigue, and rash, in addition to hypertension and QT prolongation. In addition, the utility of these systemic therapies is time-limited due to eventual tumor resistance, and neither vandetanib or cabozantenib have been shown to improve OS.[71] Acquired resistance to TKIs that target RET is likely the result of mutations that modify the RET kinase or that enable bypass signaling.[72] Specifically, there is evidence that the *RET* V804 M mutation provides a gatekeeper function that is associated with primary and acquired resistance to multikinase inhibitor treatment.[73,74] Therefore, selective RET inhibitors were screened for activity against gatekeeper mutations in development.[72]

Selective RET inhibitors were developed to achieve higher potency anti-tumor effects with less toxicity. Selpercatinib and pralsetinib are selective RET inhibitors that are FDA-approved for the management of *RET*-mutated unresectable MTC and have improved side effect profiles compared with multikinase inhibitors, likely due to less activity against VEGFR2.[75] In a phase I/II open-label trial of selpercatinib in patients with *RET*-mutant MTC with and without prior treatment with multikinase inhibitors, an objective response was observed in 69% of patients with prior vandetanib and/or cabozantinib treatment (with 86% of responses ongoing at 1 year) and 73% of patients who had not received prior targeted systemic therapy (with 91% of responses ongoing at 1 year).[76] Of note, only 12 of 531 (2%) patients treated with selpercatinib in this trial discontinued therapy due to drug-related adverse events. In updated results from the phase I/II ARROW study released in 2020, pralsetinib showed an objective response rate of 74% in treatment-naïve *RET*-mutated MTC, with a 60% objective response in patients who had previously received multikinase therapy.[77] Less than 3% of patients discontinued pralsetinib treatment due to treatment-related adverse events, which included hypertension, fatigue, and diarrhea.[75] There are other promising selective RET inhibitors currently under investigation in the management of MTC, including BOS172738[78] and TPX-0046,[79] which may lead to additional treatment options and second-line therapies that target mutations that lead to resistance to other TKIs. On the basis of these data showing good efficacy and better side effect profiles, patients with symptomatic or progressive metastatic MTC should be treated with selpercatinib or pralsetinib.

As a result of exceptional responses observed with targeted therapy (especially for selpercatinib and pralsetinib) in locally advanced or metastatic MTC, a clinical question that may be encountered is whether surgical resection should be performed in those patients who respond and have a persistent low-volume disease, or whether neoadjuvant therapy should be considered in those with borderline resectable MTC.[80,81] There is a phase II trial studying the neoadjuvant use of selpercatinib in locally advanced *RET*-mutated MTC that is currently recruiting patients to determine if this will improve the rate of R0 resection, PFS, and OS (NCT04759911). In addition, a currently recruiting, phase III randomized trial (NCT04211337) that will compare treatment with selpercatinib versus physician's choice of cabozantinib or vandetanib will further inform treatment strategies. Additional next steps to be addressed will include developing combination targeted therapies for common co-alterations that occur with selective and multi-kinase inhibitors used for the treatment of advanced MTC.[82]

Other Systemic Therapy

Peptide receptor radionuclide therapy (PRRT) targeting the somatostatin receptor (SSTR) was developed for the management of progressive gastroenteropancreatic and lung neuroendocrine tumors. Lutetium-177 dotatate was approved for this indication in 2018. Targeted radiotherapy has also been investigated for the treatment of advanced and progressive MTC, with a focus on SSTR and the cholecystokinin 2 receptor (CCK2R), two receptors commonly expressed on MTC cells in vitro and in vivo.[83] A systematic review of PRRT therapy in MTC reported on the results of 186 patients treated with PRRT targeting the SSTR with lutetium-177 and yttrium-90.[83] With heterogeneous evaluation and reporting of results within studies, they described radiographic responses, with 44 out of 117 (37.6%) of patients showing progressive disease, 64 (54.7%) having stable disease, and 6 (5.1%) patients showing a partial response. Adverse effects of therapy requiring discontinuation of PRRT occurred in 2 out of 154 (1.3%) patients with available data due to kidney toxicity. A meta-analysis of PRRT in four studies with 98 MTC patients with any uptake on SSTR scintigraphy or PET/CT that was published in 2020 reported an objective response rate of 8.5%, a disease control rate of 54%, and a serious adverse event rate of 2.8%.[84] On the basis of these early data and experience, PRRT is a potential treatment option that can be considered under investigational protocols for patients with advanced, progressive MTC and uptake on SSTR-based imaging studies.

Immune-based therapies are being investigated as additional treatment options for patients with advanced thyroid cancers, including MTC. A recent study looking at tissue from 46 patients with MTC found organized immune infiltration in 49% and 90% of primary and metastatic tumors and low-level *PD-L1* expression in a subset of patients, suggesting MTC to be an immunologically active tumor that has the potential to be treated with immune checkpoint blockade or T-cell therapies targeting tumor-associated proteins.[85,86] Small studies have shown partial responses in a subset of patients who received tumor vaccines developed to stimulate dendritic cells to present tumor-associated antigens (CEA, calcitonin, and tumor lysate), resulting in cytotoxic T cells directed at MTC cells.[87–89] Although there are clinical trials that have included or are recruiting patients with MTC for investigational protocols involving anti-PD1 and anti-CTLA4 therapies and tumor vaccines,[86] there are currently no clinical trial data to guide the use of immunotherapy in patients with MTC.

SURVEILLANCE

Following initial surgical management, patients with MTC should have biochemical testing to determine the likelihood of persistent disease. Curative surgery should result in an undetectable calcitonin and CEA within the normal range. However, the time that it takes for these tumor markers to fall post-operatively is dependent on the degree of elevation preoperatively and the burden of nodal disease. Machens and colleagues[90] recently showed in a cohort of 395 patients with MTC that time-to-normalization of calcitonin in node-negative patients was dependent on preoperative basal calcitonin levels (taking a mean of 3.7 days with calcitonin 10 to 100 pg/mL and a mean of 57.7 days with calcitonin >1000 pg/mL), whereas time-to-normalization in node-positive patients was dependent on the number of nodal metastases (mean of 5.2 days in patients with 1 to 5 nodes vs mean 57.1 days in patients with >10 nodes). Therefore, we recommend testing calcitonin and CEA as soon as 1 month following surgery in node-negative patients or 3 months postoperatively in patients with a larger burden of disease to ensure tumor marker measurement is made at the postoperative nadir and can inform further surveillance protocols.

For patients with undetectable calcitonin, the ATA guidelines recommend surveillance with physical examination and serum calcitonin and CEA levels twice yearly for two years and then yearly, in addition to ultrasound at 3 to 6 months postoperatively to establish a baseline for ongoing surveillance.[1] Patients with evidence of persistent disease based on elevated postoperative calcitonin levels warrant further evaluation and management depending on the degree of elevation. Patients with low-level postoperative calcitonin elevation (<150 pg/mL), should undergo evaluation with ultrasound and cross-sectional CT or MR with contrast to evaluate for locoregional nodal disease in the neck that can be addressed surgically. If ipsilateral and contralateral lateral neck dissections were not performed with initial surgical intervention, this should be completed. Patients with more significant elevations in calcitonin should have imaging to evaluate for distant metastases and serial calcitonin and CEA measurements to calculate doubling times to assess the likelihood of disease progression.

TREATMENT FOR PERSISTENT OR RECURRENT DISEASE

To determine the best management strategy for persistent or recurrent MTC, it is necessary to assess the following:

- Can the disease be localized and, if so, is it locoregional or distant?
- Burden of disease
- Anticipated or documented rate of disease progression
- *RET* mutational status
- Associated symptoms

The risks and benefits of reoperative neck dissections should be weighed cautiously in patients with persistent or recurrent disease, especially when calcitonin levels are >1000 and distant disease is likely, given the risks of hypoparathyroidism or recurrent laryngeal nerve injury are elevated in this setting and may adversely affect the quality of life. Active surveillance may be appropriate in this setting, ensuring local structures would not be threatened by progressive disease. Although some studies suggest biochemical cure is rarely achieved in the reoperative setting,[91] others have reported long-term cures for a subset of patients, so decisions about reoperation should be made considering individual imaging and biochemical data.[92,93] In the setting of limited metastatic disease, active surveillance may be appropriate, with enlarging or symptomatic lesions addressed locally with surgical resection, EBRT, or local embolization or radiofrequency ablation.

The initiation of systemic targeted therapy is generally delayed until patients develop progressive or symptomatic locally advanced or metastatic disease that cannot be addressed with local therapies, given patients are likely to develop treatment resistance over time. Mutational analysis of progressive disease should be performed to determine *RET* mutation status or other targetable mutations that will dictate first-line treatment. Once *RET* mutation is confirmed, selpercatinib or pralsetinib can be initiated, with surveillance for response and disease control. Patients without *RET* mutations can be treated with a multikinase inhibitor (ie, vandetanib or cabozantinib). Patients with progressive disease following initial targeted therapy should seek additional treatment as part of a clinical trial, given there are additional agents and novel therapies currently under investigation for the management of MTC.

Significant elevations in calcitonin, especially in the setting of MTC liver metastases, can lead to systemic symptoms that can be bothersome to patients, including diarrhea and facial flushing. Symptom improvement can be achieved with a high-fiber diet and anti-motility agents or, in patients with intractable symptoms, somatostatin analogs and/or chemoembolization of liver metastases.[94,95] In addition, some MTCs produce ACTH, causing ectopic Cushing's syndrome, which usually occurs in advanced-stage MTC and is associated with a poor prognosis.[96,97] Depending on the severity of the hypercortisolism, patients can be trialed on adrenal enzyme inhibitors (ie, ketoconazole or metyrapone). If the ectopic Cushing's syndrome is associated with a progressive disease that warrants the initiation of systemic therapy, they may improve with targeted therapy with selective or multikinase inhibitors.[97] However, bilateral adrenalectomy may be necessary for the ultimate control of hypercortisolism in patients who do not respond to other management strategies.

SUMMARY

The management of patients with MTC continues to evolve based on expanding evidence related to biochemical testing and the appropriate extent of surgical intervention, advances in cross-sectional and nuclear medicine imaging techniques, and, most notably, the approval of the selective RET inhibitors selpercatinib and pralsetinib. These systemic targeted therapies are likely to greatly improve the management of patients with locally advanced or metastatic disease. Ongoing research determines how these new drugs can best be used to improve the care of patients with MTC.

DISCLOSURE

The authors have nothing to disclose.

REFERENCES

1. Wells SA, Asa SL, Dralle H, et al. Revised American Thyroid Association Guidelines for the Management of Medullary Thyroid Carcinoma. Thyroid 2015;25(6): 567–610.
2. Fussey JM, Vaidya B, Kim D, et al. The role of molecular genetics in the clinical management of sporadic medullary thyroid carcinoma: A systematic review. Clin Endocrinol 2019;91(6):697–707.
3. Vuong HG, Odate T, Ngo HTT, et al. Clinical significance of RET and RAS mutations in sporadic medullary thyroid carcinoma: a meta-analysis. Endocrine-Related Cancer 2018;25(6):633–41.
4. Moura MM, Cavaco BM, Leite V. RAS proto-oncogene in medullary thyroid carcinoma. Endocr Relat Cancer 2015;22(5):R235–52.
5. Salvatore D, Santoro M, Schlumberger M. The importance of the RET gene in thyroid cancer and therapeutic implications. Nat Rev Endocrinol 2021;17(5):296–306.
6. Pasini B, Borrello MG, Greco A, et al. Loss of function effect of RET mutations causing Hirschsprung disease. Nat Genet 1995;10(1):35–40.

7. Santoro M, Carlomagno F, Romano A, et al. Activation of RET as a dominant trans-forming gene by germline mutations of MEN2A and MEN2B. Science (New York, NY) 1995;267(5196):381–3.
8. Romei C, Ciampi R, Elisei R. A comprehensive overview of the role of the RET proto-oncogene in thyroid carcinoma. Nat Rev Endocrinol 2016;12(4):192–202.
9. Maciel RMB, Maia AL. GLOBAL ENDOCRINOLOGY: Geographical variation in the profile of RET variants in patients with medullary thyroid cancer: a compre-hensive review. Eur J Endocrinol 2021;186(1):R15–30.
10. Machens A, Niccoli-Sire P, Hoegel J, et al. Early malignant progression of hered-itary medullary thyroid cancer. N Engl J Med 2003;349(16):1517–25.
11. Skinner MA, Moley JA, Dilley WG, et al. Prophylactic thyroidectomy in multiple endocrine neoplasia type 2A. N Engl J Med 2005;353(11):1105–13.
12. Castinetti F, Qi X-P, Walz MK, et al. Outcomes of adrenal-sparing surgery or total adrenalectomy in phaeochromocytoma associated with multiple endocrine neoplasia type 2: an international retrospective population-based study. Lancet Oncol 2014;15(6):648–55.
13. Kebebew E, Ituarte PH, Siperstein AE, et al. Medullary thyroid carcinoma: clinical characteristics, treatment, prognostic factors, and a comparison of staging sys-tems. Cancer 2000;88(5):1139–48.
14. Kebebew E, Tresler PA, Siperstein AE, et al. Normal thyroid pathology in patients undergoing thyroidectomy for finding a RET gene germline mutation: a report of three cases and review of the literature. Thyroid 1999;9(2):127–31.
15. Machens A, Elwerr M, Lorenz K, et al. Long-term outcome of prophylactic thyroid-ectomy in children carrying RET germline mutations. Br J Surg 2018;105(2): e150–7.
16. Moura MM, Cavaco BM, Pinto AE, et al. High Prevalence of RAS Mutations in RET-Negative Sporadic Medullary Thyroid Carcinomas. J Clin Endocrinol Metab 2011;96(5):E863–8.
17. Pusztaszeri MP, Bongiovanni M, Faquin WC. Update on the cytologic and molec-ular features of medullary thyroid carcinoma. Adv Anat Pathol 2014;21(1):26–35.
18. Dyhdalo KS, Chute DJ. Barriers to the recognition of medullary thyroid carcinoma on FNA: Implications relevant to the new American Thyroid Association guide-lines. Cancer Cytopathology 2018;126(6):397–405.
19. Verbeek HH, de Groot JWB, Sluiter WJ, et al. Calcitonin testing for detection of medullary thyroid cancer in people with thyroid nodules. Cochrane Database Syst Rev 2020;(3):1–98.
20. Wang L, Kou H, Chen W, et al. The diagnostic value of ultrasound in medullary thyroid carcinoma: a comparison with computed tomography. Technology Can-cer Res Treat 2020;19. 1533033820905832.
21. Valderrabano P, Klippenstein DL, Tourtelot JB, et al. New American Thyroid Asso-ciation sonographic patterns for thyroid nodules perform well in medullary thyroid carcinoma: institutional experience, systematic review, and meta-analysis. Thy-roid 2016;26(8):1093–100.
22. Yun G, Kim YK, Choi SI, et al. Medullary thyroid carcinoma: application of thyroid imaging reporting and data system (TI-RADS) classification. Endocrine 2018; 61(2):285–92.
23. Giraudet AL, Vanel D, Leboulleux S, et al. Imaging medullary thyroid carcinoma with persistent elevated calcitonin levels. J Clin Endocrinol Metab 2007;92(11): 4185–90.
24. Dromain C, de Baere T, Lumbroso J, et al. Detection of liver metastases from endocrine tumors: a prospective comparison of somatostatin receptor

scintigraphy, computed tomography, and magnetic resonance imaging. J Clin Oncol 2005;23(1):70–8.
25. Lee S-W, Shim SR, Jeong SY, et al. Comparison of 5 different PET radiopharmaceuticals for the detection of recurrent medullary thyroid carcinoma: a network meta-analysis. Clin Nucl Med 2020;45(5):341–8.
26. Treglia G, Castaldi P, Villani MF, et al. Comparison of 18F-DOPA, 18F-FDG and 68Ga-somatostatin analogue PET/CT in patients with recurrent medullary thyroid carcinoma. Eur J Nucl Med Mol Imaging 2012;39(4):569–80.
27. Golubić AT, Pasini Nemir E, Žuvić M, et al. The value of 18F-DOPA PET/CT in patients with medullary thyroid carcinoma and increased calcitonin values. Nucl Med Commun 2017;38(7):636–41.
28. Treglia G, Cocciolillo F, Di Nardo F, et al. Detection rate of recurrent medullary thyroid carcinoma using fluorine-18 dihydroxyphenylalanine positron emission tomography: a meta-analysis. Acad Radiol 2012;19(10):1290–9.
29. Ong SC, Schöder H, Patel SG, et al. Diagnostic accuracy of 18F-FDG PET in restaging patients with medullary thyroid carcinoma and elevated calcitonin levels. J Nucl Med 2007;48(4):501–7.
30. Treglia G, Tamburello A, Giovanella L. Detection rate of somatostatin receptor PET in patients with recurrent medullary thyroid carcinoma: a systematic review and a meta-analysis. Hormones 2017;16(4):362–72.
31. Giovanella L, Treglia G, Iakovou I, et al. EANM practice guideline for PET/CT imaging in medullary thyroid carcinoma. Eur J Nucl Med Mol Imaging 2020;47(1): 61–77.
32. Castinetti F, Taïeb D. Positron Emission Tomography Imaging in Medullary Thyroid Carcinoma: Time for Reappraisal? Thyroid 2021;31(2):151–5.
33. Perros P, Boelaert K, Colley S, et al. Guidelines for the management of thyroid cancer. Clin Endocrinol 2014;81(s1):1–122.
34. Patel KN, Yip L, Lubitz CC, et al. The American Association of Endocrine Surgeons guidelines for the definitive surgical management of thyroid disease in adults. Ann Surg 2020;271(3):e21–93.
35. Machens A, Dralle H. Biomarker-based risk stratification for previously untreated medullary thyroid cancer. J Clin Endocrinol Metab 2010;95(6):2655–63.
36. Machens A, Lorenz K, Weber F, et al. Exceptionality of Distant Metastasis in Node-Negative Hereditary and Sporadic Medullary Thyroid Cancer: Lessons Learned. J Clin Endocrinol Metab 2021;106(8):e2968–79. https://doi.org/10.1210/clinem/dgab214.
37. McMullen C, Rocke D, Freeman J. Complications of bilateral neck dissection in thyroid cancer from a single high-volume center. JAMA Otolaryngology–Head Neck Surg 2017;143(4):376–81.
38. Sosa JA, Tuggle CT, Wang TS, et al. Clinical and economic outcomes of thyroid and parathyroid surgery in children. J Clin Endocrinol Metab 2008;93(8): 3058–65.
39. Fersht N, Vini L, A'hern R, et al. The role of radiotherapy in the management of elevated calcitonin after surgery for medullary thyroid cancer. Thyroid 2001; 11(12):1161–8.
40. Brierley J, Tsang R, Simpson W, et al. Medullary thyroid cancer: analyses of survival and prognostic factors and the role of radiation therapy in local control. Thyroid 1996;6(4):305–10.
41. Rowell NP. The role of external beam radiotherapy in the management of medullary carcinoma of the thyroid: A systematic review. Radiother Oncol 2019;136: 113–20.

42. Wu LT, Averbuch SD, Ball DW, et al. Treatment of advanced medullary thyroid carcinoma with a combination of cyclophosphamide, vincristine, and dacarbazine. Cancer 1994;73(2):432–6.

43. Nocera M, Baudin E, Pellegriti G, et al. Treatment of advanced medullary thyroid cancer with an alternating combination of doxorubicin-streptozocin and 5 FU-dacarbazine. Br J Cancer 2000;83(6):715–8.

44. Edge SbAJCoC. AJCC cancer staging manual. 8th edition. Chicago, IL: Springer; 2017.

45. Esfandiari NH, Hughes DT, Yin H, et al. The Effect of Extent of Surgery and Number of Lymph Node Metastases on Overall Survival in Patients with Medullary Thyroid Cancer. J Clin Endocrinol Metab 2014;99(2):448–54.

46. Adam MA, Thomas S, Roman SA, et al. Rethinking the Current American Joint Committee on Cancer TNM Staging System for Medullary Thyroid Cancer. JAMA Surg 2017;152(9):869–76.

47. Machens A, Dralle H. Prognostic impact of N staging in 715 medullary thyroid cancer patients: proposal for a revised staging system. Ann Surg 2013;257(2):323–9.

48. Wang Z, Tang C, Wang Y, et al. Inclusion of the Number of Metastatic Lymph Nodes in the Staging System for Medullary Thyroid Cancer: Validating a Modified AJCC TNM Staging System. Thyroid 2022. https://doi.org/10.1089/thy.2021.0571.

49. Yang JH, Lindsey SC, Camacho CP, et al. Integration of a postoperative calcitonin measurement into an anatomical staging system improves initial risk stratification in medullary thyroid cancer. Clin Endocrinol 2015;83(6):938–42.

50. Barbet J, Campion Lc, Kraeber-Bodéré Fo, et al. Prognostic Impact of Serum Calcitonin and Carcinoembryonic Antigen Doubling-Times in Patients with Medullary Thyroid Carcinoma. J Clin Endocrinol Metab 2005;90(11):6077–84.

51. Alencar R, Kendler DB, Andrade F, et al. CA19-9 as a predictor of worse clinical outcome in medullary thyroid carcinoma. Eur Thyroid J 2019;8(4):186–91.

52. Xu B, Fuchs TL, Ahmadi S, et al. International Medullary Thyroid Carcinoma Grading System: A Validated Grading System for Medullary Thyroid Carcinoma. J Clin Oncol 2022;40(1):96–104.

53. Saad MF, Ordonez NG, Rashid RK, et al. Medullary carcinoma of the thyroid. A study of the clinical features and prognostic factors in 161 patients. Medicine 1984;63(6):319–42.

54. Sahli ZT, Canner JK, Zeiger MA, et al. Association between age and disease specific mortality in medullary thyroid cancer. Am J Surg 2021;221(2):478–84.

55. Miyauchi A, Onishi T, Morimoto S, et al. Relation of doubling time of plasma calcitonin levels to prognosis and recurrence of medullary thyroid carcinoma. Ann Surg 1984;199(4):461.

56. Yeh T, Yeung M, Sherman EJ, et al. Structural doubling time predicts overall survival in patients with medullary thyroid cancer in patients with rapidly progressive metastatic medullary thyroid cancer treated with molecular targeted therapies. Thyroid 2020;30(8):1112–9.

57. Elisei R, Lorusso L, Romei C, et al. Medullary Thyroid Cancer Secreting Carbohydrate Antigen 19-9 (Ca 19-9): A Fatal Case Report. J Clin Endocrinol Metab 2013;98(9):3550–4.

58. Milman S, Whitney KD, Fleischer N. Metastatic medullary thyroid cancer presenting with elevated levels of CA 19-9 and CA 125. Thyroid 2011;21(8):913–6.

59. Vierbuchen M, Larena A, Schröder S, et al. Blood group antigen expression in medullary carcinoma of the thyroid. An immunohistochemical study on the

occurrence of type 1 chain-derived antigens. Virchows Arch B Cell Pathol Incl Mol Pathol 1992;62(2):79–88.

60. Lorusso L, Romei C, Piaggi P, et al. Ca19.9 Positivity and Doubling Time Are Prognostic Factors of Mortality in Patients with Advanced Medullary Thyroid Cancer with No Evidence of Structural Disease Progression According to Response Evaluation Criteria in Solid Tumors. Thyroid 2021;31(7):1050–5.

61. Rodríguez-Antona C, Pallares J, Montero-Conde C, et al. Overexpression and activation of EGFR and VEGFR2 in medullary thyroid carcinomas is related to metastasis. Endocrine-Related Cancer 2010;17(1):7–16.

62. Wells SA Jr, Robinson BG, Gagel RF, et al. Vandetanib in patients with locally advanced or metastatic medullary thyroid cancer: a randomized, double-blind phase III trial. J Clin Oncol 2012;30(2):134.

63. Elisei R, Schlumberger MJ, Müller SP, et al. Cabozantinib in progressive medullary thyroid cancer. J Clin Oncol 2013;31(29):3639.

64. Schlumberger M, Elisei R, Müller S, et al. Overall survival analysis of EXAM, a phase III trial of cabozantinib in patients with radiographically progressive medullary thyroid carcinoma. Ann Oncol 2017;28(11):2813–9.

65. Schlumberger M, Jarzab B, Cabanillas ME, et al. A Phase II Trial of the Multitargeted Tyrosine Kinase Inhibitor Lenvatinib (E7080) in Advanced Medullary Thyroid CancerPhase II Trial of Lenvatinib in Medullary Thyroid Cancer. Clin Cancer Res 2016;22(1):44–53.

66. Matrone A, Prete A, Nervo A, et al. Lenvatinib as a salvage therapy for advanced metastatic medullary thyroid cancer. J Endocrinological Invest 2021;44(10):2139–51.

67. Lam ET, Ringel MD, Kloos RT, et al. Phase II clinical trial of sorafenib in metastatic medullary thyroid cancer. J Clin Oncol 2010;28(14):2323.

68. De Souza J, Busaidy N, Zimrin A, et al. Phase II trial of sunitinib in medullary thyroid cancer (MTC). J Clin Oncol 2010;28(15_suppl):5504.

69. Ravaud A, de la Fouchardière C, Caron P, et al. A multicenter phase II study of sunitinib in patients with locally advanced or metastatic differentiated, anaplastic or medullary thyroid carcinomas: mature data from the THYSU study. Eur J Cancer 2017;76:110–7.

70. Chougnet CN, Borget I, Leboulleux S, et al. Vandetanib for the treatment of advanced medullary thyroid cancer outside a clinical trial: results from a French cohort. Thyroid 2015;25(4):386–91.

71. Kesby NL, Papachristos AJ, Gild M, et al. Outcomes of Advanced Medullary Thyroid Carcinoma in the Era of Targeted Therapy. Ann Surg Oncol 2022;29(1):64–71.

72. Subbiah V, Cote GJ. Advances in targeting RET-dependent cancers. Cancer Discov 2020;10(4):498–505.

73. Carlomagno F, Guida T, Anaganti S, et al. Disease associated mutations at valine 804 in the RET receptor tyrosine kinase confer resistance to selective kinase inhibitors. Oncogene 2004;23(36):6056–63.

74. Busaidy N, Cabanillas M, Sherman S, et al. Emergence of V804M resistance gatekeeper mutation in sporadic medullary thyroid carcinoma patients treated with TKI tyrosine kinase inhibitors. Thyroid 2017;27(Suppl 1):A168.

75. Subbiah V, Yang D, Velcheti V, et al. State-of-the-art strategies for targeting RET-dependent cancers. J Clin Oncol 2020;38(11):1209.

76. Wirth LJ, Sherman E, Robinson B, et al. Efficacy of Selpercatinib in RET-Altered Thyroid Cancers. New Engl J Med 2020;383(9):825–35.

77. Subbiah V, Hu MI-N, Gainor JF, et al. Clinical activity of the RET inhibitor pralsetinib (BLU-667) in patients with RET fusion+ solid tumors. J Clin Oncol 2020; 38(15 Suppl):109.

78. Schoffski P, Aftimos PG, Massard C, et al. A phase I study of BOS172738 in patients with advanced solid tumors with RET gene alterations including non-small cell lung cancer and medullary thyroid cancer. Am Soc Clin Oncol 2019.

79. Drilon A, Rogers E, Zhai D, et al. TPX-0046 is a novel and potent RET/SRC inhibitor for RET-driven cancers. Ann Oncol 2019;30:v190–1.

80. Jozaghi Y, Zafereo M, Williams MD, et al. Neoadjuvant selpercatinib for advanced medullary thyroid cancer. Head & Neck 2021;43(1):E7–12.

81. Grasic Kuhar C, Lozar T, Besic N, et al. Outcome of Patients with Locally Advanced Metastatic Medullary Thyroid Cancer and Induction Therapy with Tyrosine Kinase Inhibitors in Slovenia. Adv Ther 2021;38(12):5684–99.

82. Kurzrock R. Selpercatinib Aimed at RET-Altered Cancers. New Engl J Med 2020; 383(9):868–9.

83. Grossrubatscher E, Fanciulli G, Pes L, et al. Advances in the management of medullary thyroid carcinoma: focus on peptide receptor radionuclide therapy. J Clin Med 2020;9(11):3507.

84. Lee DY, Kim Y-i. Peptide Receptor Radionuclide Therapy in Patients With Differentiated Thyroid Cancer: A Meta-analysis. Clin Nucl Med 2020;45(8):604–10.

85. Pozdeyev N, Erickson TA, Zhang L, et al. Comprehensive immune profiling of medullary thyroid cancer. Thyroid 2020;30(9):1263–79.

86. French JD. Immunotherapy for advanced thyroid cancers—rationale, current advances and future strategies. Nat Rev Endocrinol 2020;16(11):629–41.

87. Bachleitner-Hofmann T, Friedl J, Hassler M, et al. Pilot trial of autologous dendritic cells loaded with tumor lysate (s) from allogeneic tumor cell lines in patients with metastatic medullary thyroid carcinoma. Oncol Rep 2009;21(6):1585–92.

88. Schott M, Feldkamp J, Klucken M, et al. Calcitonin-specific antitumor immunity in medullary thyroid carcinoma following dendritic cell vaccination. Cancer Immunol Immunother 2002;51(11):663–8.

89. Schott M, Seissler J, Lettmann M, et al. Immunotherapy for medullary thyroid carcinoma by dendritic cell vaccination. J Clin Endocrinol Metab 2001;86(10): 4965–9.

90. Machens A, Lorenz K, Dralle H. Time to calcitonin normalization after surgery for node-negative and node-positive medullary thyroid cancer. J Br Surg 2019; 106(4):412–8.

91. Van Heerden J, Grant CS, Gharib H, et al. Long-term course of patients with persistent hypercalcitoninemia after apparent curative primary surgery for medullary thyroid carcinoma. Ann Surg 1990;212(4):395.

92. Fialkowski E, DeBenedetti M, Moley J. Long-term outcome of reoperations for medullary thyroid carcinoma. World J Surg 2008;32(5):754–65.

93. Kebebew E, Kikuchi S, Duh QY, et al. Long-term results of reoperation and localizing studies in patients with persistent or recurrent medullary thyroid cancer. Arch Surg 2000;135(8):895–901.

94. Fromigue J, De Baere T, Baudin E, et al. Chemoembolization for liver metastases from medullary thyroid carcinoma. J Clin Endocrinol Metab 2006;91(7):2496–9.

95. Lorenz K, Brauckhoff M, Behrmann C, et al. Selective arterial chemoembolization for hepatic metastases from medullary thyroid carcinoma. Surgery 2005;138(6):986–93.

96. Koehler VF, Fuss CT, Berr CM, et al. Medullary thyroid cancer with ectopic Cushing's syndrome: A multicentre case series. Clin Endocrinol 2022;96(6):847–56.

97. Corsello A, RAMUNNO V, Locantore P, et al. Medullary thyroid cancer with ectopic Cushing's syndrome: a case report and systematic review of detailed cases from the literature. Thyroid 2022;(ja).

A Nomogram for Relapse/ Death and Contemplating Adjuvant Therapy for Parathyroid Carcinoma

Angelica M. Silva-Figueroa, MD, MEd[a,b,*]

KEYWORDS

- Parathyroid carcinoma • Parathyroid cancer • Parathyroid neoplasms • Prognosis
- Nomograms • Molecular targeted therapy • Next-generation sequencing
- Immunotherapy

INTRODUCTION

Parathyroid carcinoma (PC) is a rare endocrine disease. Until 2001, the annual incidence was 1 to 3 people per 10 million; in the last decade, however, its annual incidence in the United States and Asia has increased to approximately 10 people per 10 million.[1–4] Lee and colleagues suggest that this increased incidence is the result of 2002 National Institutes of Health guidelines on parathyroidectomy in asymptomatic patients with hyperparathyroidism identified by screening for hypercalcemia.[1,5–7]

Various clinical and biochemical findings can raise suspicion of the presence of a PC. These include palpable cervical mass, parathyroid gland >30 mm, moderate-to-severe hypercalcemia, significantly elevated parathyroid hormone (PTH) levels (three to five times the limit of normal), and intraoperative observation of adhesions to surrounding tissues (thyroid, muscle, esophagus, and laryngeal nerve).[7–10] However, PC can be difficult to distinguish from other etiologic causes of hyperparathyroidism during preoperative and intraoperative diagnosis because the previously mentioned parameters are not categorically present. Thus, the unequivocal histopathological presentation is required to confirm the PC diagnosis.

Currently, the histologic diagnosis of PC is restricted to those parathyroid tumors that show one of the following: angioinvasion, lymphatic invasion, perineural or intraneural invasion, local malignant invasion into other anatomic structures, or histologically/cytologically documented metastatic disease.[11] In 2022, the World Health Organization (WHO) applied histopathological criteria and defined the roles of ancillary techniques for the diagnosis of PC. Biomarkers in the new WHO classification for the differential diagnosis of PC included are; APC, RB, E-cadherin, p27, Bcl-2a, mdm-2,

[a] Universidad Finis Terrae, School of Medicine, Chile; [b] Service of Surgery, Department of Head and Neck Surgery, Hospital Barros Luco Trudeau, Santiago, Chile
* Universidad Finis Terrae, School of Medicine, Providencia, Santiago 7501015, Chile.
E-mail address: angelica.silva@uft.cl

Surg Oncol Clin N Am 32 (2023) 251–269
https://doi.org/10.1016/j.soc.2022.10.003
1055-3207/23/© 2022 Elsevier Inc. All rights reserved.
surgonc.theclinics.com

5-hmC, PGP9.5, galectin-3, and hTERT; p53 overexpression; and an increased Ki-67 labeling index (often >5%).[11] Although none of these biomarkers alone is definitive, their use in combination is recommended for complex cases.

The gold standard treatment of PC is complete tumor resection with R0 margins. Patients with PC have a 5-year overall survival (OS) of 83% to 91%, and a 10-year OS of 49% to 88%. However, more than half of PC patients will have locally or distant recurrent disease within 5 years of the first surgical intervention,[1,10,12] usually between years 2 and 5 (42% to 72% of patients), and the median OS is 14 years.[13–18] Surgical resection remains the primary therapeutic intervention for patients with multiple locoregional recurrences because both radiotherapy and chemotherapy are not effective by themselves or as adjuvants.[19] Effective therapeutic options are scarce when distant metastases develop, and death results from a lethal course of uncontrollable hypercalcemia.

Despite the rise in incidence of PC in the last decade, PC remains a low-frequency malignant neoplasm that is heterogeneously reported, making it very difficult to reach consensus with validated data. A proven staging system for PC that establishes a multivariate analysis with prognostic significance is still not available, owing to the fact that it is a rare disease, and most reports are of single-institution retrospective studies or datasets from large databases with missing data for a substantial number of patients. The 8th Edition of the AJCC Staging Manual states that identifying significant prognostic factors has been a major challenge, and it proposes that a standardized TNM staging system for PC would be highly anticipated without solid evidence.[20] Thus, assigning a personalized prognosis for patients with PC and standardization of management according to the risk of relapse and death remain difficult.

Here, we review the latest findings and advances toward developing prognostic criteria to predict relapse and their potential in establishing a standardized staging system. We also review new therapeutic approaches for PC based on tumor profiling.

DISCUSSION
Staging System and Relapse

In the last 12 years, several proposals have been made for TNM-type prognostic prediction in PC (**Table 1**). One of the first proposed staging systems was published in 1999, which was based on anatomic progression and emphasized tumor size in 330 patients with PC.[21] Subsequently, Talat and Schulte, in their univariate analysis, showed that male sex (relative risk [RR] = 1.7; 95% confidence interval [CI], 1.0 to 2.7; $P < .01$), angioinvasion (RR = 4.3; 95% CI, 1.1 to 17.7; $P < .01$), and lymph node metastasis (RR = 6.2; 95% CI, 0.9 to 42.9; $P < .001$) influenced recurrence and survival rates.[16] In their study, cases were divided into groups with high risk (angioinvasion, lymph node metastasis and/or invasion of vital organs and/or distant metastasis) or low risk (capsular invasion and/or soft tissue invasion), and an increased risk of recurrence and death was detected in the high-risk group (3.5 to 7.0-fold, $P < .01$).[16] In 2012, Schulte created another staging proposal to validate the staging system that was developed in 2010 with Talat.[16,22] In this study, Schulte and colleagues[22] showed that PCs considered high risk had a lower 5-year DFS ($P < .005$ for $n = 45$) and a higher risk of tumor relapse (RR = 9.6; 95% CI, 2.4 to 38.2; $P < .0001$). The TNM cancer manual from the combined AJCC, with the UICC 8th edition 2017, has requested to collect of specific variables from PC cases to collate a sufficiently robust dataset to finalize a formal staging system[20,23,24]; validation of the prognostic significance of some variables remains incomplete, and this effort is ongoing. **Table 2** are represented the recommended variables for prospective registration in medical centers.

Table 1
Proposed TNM staging system for parathyroid carcinoma in the literature

Shaha (Saha & Shah,[21] 1999)		Talat and Schulte (Talat & Schulte,[16] 2010; Schulte et al,[22] 2012)		TNM AJCC UICC 8th Edition (Amin et al,[24] 2017)
T	Tx not defined	T	Tx not defined	T	Tx primary cannot be assessed T0 no evidence of primary tumor Tis neoplasm of uncertain malignant potential (atypical)
	T1 primary tumor < 3 cm		T1 capsular invasion		T1 localized to the parathyroid gland with extension limited to soft tissue
	T2 primary tumor > 3 cm		T2 invasion of surrounding soft tissues excluding the vital organs trachea, larynx, and esophagus		T2 direct invasion into the thyroid gland
	T3 any tumoral size with invasion of the surrounding soft tissues, that is, thyroid gland, and strap muscles.		T3 angioinvasion		T3 direct invasion into recurrent laryngeal nerve, esophagus, trachea, skeletal muscle, adjacent lymph nodes, or thymus
	T4 massive central disease invading trachea and esophagus or recurrence PC		T4 invasion of vital organs, that is, hypopharynx, trachea, esophagus, larynx, recurrent laryngeal nerve, carotid artery		T4 direct invasion into major blood vessel or spine
N	Nx not defined	N	Nx not assessed or unknown	N	Nx regional lymph nodes cannot be assessed
	N0 no lymph nodes disease		N0 No lymph nodes disease		N0 no lymph nodes disease
	N1 lymph nodes disease		N1 lymph nodes disease		N1a metastasis to level VI or level VII N1b metastasis to unilateral, bilateral, or contralateral cervical, or retropharyngeal nodes
M	Mx not defined	M	Mx not assessed or unknown	M	Mx distant metastasis cannot be assessed
	M0 no distant metastasis		M0 no distant metastasis		M0 no distant metastasis
	M1 evidence of distant metastasis		M1 evidence of distant metastasis		M1 distant metastasis

(continued on next page)

	Table 1 *(continued)*		
	Shaha (Saha & Shah,[21] 1999)	**Talat and Schulte (Talat & Schulte,[16] 2010; Schulte et al,[22] 2012)**	**TNM AJCC UICC 8th Edition (Amin et al,[24] 2017)**
Stage	I T1N0M0 II T2N0M0 IIIa T3N0M0 IIIb T4N0M0 IIIc any T, N1M0 IV any T, any N,M1	*Stage* I T1 or T2 N0M0 II T3N0M0 III any T, N1M0 or T4 IV any N, M1	*Stage* There are not enough data to propose anatomic stage and prognostic groups for PC.
		High and low risk Low Capsular invasion combined with invasion of surrounding soft tissue High Vascular invasion and/or lymph node metastases and/or invasion of vital organs and/or distant metastases	

Prognostic Factors for Survival and Relapse

We comprehensively reviewed the literature on studies in PC with an analysis of survival and relapse over the last 7 years, and we included multicenter studies, population databases (NCDB and SEER), countries' national health insurance, tertiary-referral cancer hospitals, and studies with innovative contributions on survival analysis in PC. In this article, we review the most consistently reported prognostic host factors, tumor and tumoral microenvironment factors that affect the clinical course of PC (**Table 3**).

Host-independent factors

Age. Since 2010, advanced age has been considered a critical factor in predicting OS in patients with PC,[16] and this has been extensively validated in large databases for multivariate and univariate analyses over the last 2 years. A study by Zhu and colleagues[25] of 193 patients with PC showed that patients aged $\geq$50 years had a significantly lower OS (hazard ratio [HR] = 2.37, P = .004) without any effect on DFS. Subsequently, Leonard-Muralli and colleagues[26] gathered information from 555 patients with PC using the NCDB, a database that captures approximately 70% of patients diagnosed annually with cancer in the United States in approximately 1,500 hospitals. Their multivariate analysis showed that age >75 years (HR = 2.87; 95% CI, 1.42 to 577; P = .003) was associated with worse OS. That same year, a multivariate analysis by Kong and colleagues[3] of 255 patients with PC from the Korean National Health Insurance Services database, which covers approximately 97.2% of Korean residents in all age groups, showed that patients with baseline age $\geq$50 years had 2.75 times higher risk of mortality than younger patients (95% CI, 1.19 to 6.38; P = .018).

In 2022, three studies were published simultaneously that used the SEER database, which covers 28% of the US population.[27–29] Quian and colleagues[27] found that age >70 years (HR = 3.55; 95% CI, 1.07 to 11.78; P = .039) is an independent factor

Table 2
Recommended variables for prospective registration to create a standardized staging system in parathyroid carcinoma

Registry Data Collection	
Variables	Criteria
Patients factors	
Age at diagnosis	
Gender	
Race	
Genetic mutations	
Tumor factors	
Size of primary tumor in millimeters	
Location of primary tumor	Left or right and superior (upper) or inferior (lower)
Invasion into surrounding tissue	Present or absent
Distant metastasis	
Number of lymph nodes removed	By level
Number of lymph nodes positive	By level
Weight of primary tumor	In milligram
Time to recurrence	Months
Biochemical and histologic Factors	
Highest preoperative calcium	mg/dL
Highest preoperative parathyroid hormone	pg/mL
Lymphovascular invasion	Present or absent
Grade	Low or high[a]
Ki 67 index	%
Mitotic rate	
Solid or trabecular growth pattern	
Tumor necrosis	Present or absent

[a] *PC low grade*: round monomorphic nuclei with only mild-to-moderate nuclear size variation, indistinct characteristics resembling those of normal parathyroid or of adenoma; *PC high grade*: show several discrete confluent areas with nuclear changes with pleomorphism, with a nuclear size variation > 4:1; prominent nuclear membrane irregularities; chromatin alterations, hyperchromasia or margination of chromatin; and prominent nucleoli.

predicting increased risk of cancer-specific death on PC. Ullah and colleagues[28] evaluated 5-year survival in a multivariate analysis and showed that age >40 years was an independent risk factor for mortality ($P < .001$). A multivariate analysis by Tao and colleagues,[29] designed to create a predictive nomogram for OS and CSS, identified age >66 years as an independent factor predicting worse OS in 342 patients with PC (HR = 3.26; 95% CI: 1.87 to 5.69; $P < .001$). An additional notable study of 733 patients with PC, published in 2015 by Asare and colleagues,[5] showed that, for each year increase in age, there was an associated 6% increase in the risk of death when adjustments were made for nodal status, sex, tumor size, and extent of resection (HR = 1.06; 95% CI, 1.05 to 1.07; $P < .0001$).

It is essential to consider age-related findings in the context that older patients tend to have worse general physiologic conditions, which leads to a higher incidence of postoperative complications, prolonged postoperative stay, and recurrence.[29,30]

Table 3
Host, tumor, and tumoral microenvironment factors that negatively affect the survival of patients with parathyroid carcinoma reported in the last 7 years in the literature

Prognostic Factors	Survival Effect Reported	References
Host factors		
Age	≥50 y ↓ Overall Survival >75 y ↓ Overall Survival ≥50 y ↑ Mortality rate >70 y ↓ Cancer-specific survival >40 y ↑ Mortality rate >66 years ↓ Overall Survival	Kong et al.[3], Zhu [25], Leonard-Murali et al.[26], Qian et al.[27], Ullah et al.[28], Tao et al.[29]
Gender	Male gender ↑ Mortality rate	Asare et al.[5], Wang et al.[32]
Biochemical factors		
Serum Calcium	>15 mg/dL ↓ Recurrence-free survival And ↑ Mortality rate	Silva-Figueroa et al.[34], Xue et al.[35]
PTH levels	>700 pg/ml ↓ Cancer-specific survival	Machens[36]
Tumor factors and invasion		
Tumor size	>40 mm ↑ Risk of death >30, 35, and 40 mm ↓ Cancer-specific survival >32 mm ↑ Risk of distant Metastasis >41 mm ↓ Overall survival	Asare et al.[5], Lo et al.[4], Asare et al.[8], Qian et al.[27], Ullah et al.[28], Tao et al.[29], Sun et al.[37]
Angioinvasion	Positive ↑ Recurrence, death, and ↓ recurrence-free survival	Talet[16], Schulte et al.[22], Silva-Figueroa et al.[34], Xue et al.[35], Villar-del-Moral et al.[40]
Distant metastasis (M)	M(+) ↓ Cancer-specific survival M(+) ↓ 5-y Overall Survival Bone M(+) ↑ Risk of distant metastasis	Lo et al.[4], Asare et al.[5], Wei et al.[38], Tsai et al.[45]
Tumoral microenvironment and Biomarkers		
Parafibromin staining	Negative ↑ Risk of recurrence/metastasis Negative ↑ Risk of death	Zhu[25,a], Hu et al.[31]
CD8	(Low) cell density ↑ Risk of relapse and ↓ Overall survival	Hu et al.[53]
CD163	(High) cell density ↑ Risk of relapse	Hu et al.[53]

[a] Meta-analysis.

Furthermore, as in other cancers, comprehensive perioperative and long-term geriatric management could improve the quality and survival of patients with PC.

Sex. Owing to inconsistencies among studies,[1] no consensus has been reached on the role of sex on PC prognosis.[5,31] In their NCDB multivariate analysis, Asare and colleagues[5] showed that males with PC had a 67% higher risk of death than females (HR = 1.67; 95% CI, 1.24 to 2.25; P = .0008). Subsequently, Wang and colleagues,[32] using the three major Chinese population databases (VIP Journal Integration Platform,

China Knowledge Resource Integrated Database, and Wanfang Data), evaluated prognostic factors associated with 5- and 10-year DFS and DSS rates in 234 patients with PC and showed that males had a higher mortality rate than females ($P = .040$).

Tumor and biochemical factors

Unfortunately, population registry systems do not record complete clinicopathological information, such as recurrence, calcium, PTH levels, and individual molecular factors. That is why the SEER database, for example, has not found these factors to facilitate multivariate analyses.[33]

Serum calcium and parathyroid hormone. In the risk stratification created in 2017 for PC, the primary endpoint was RFS rate,[34] because OS is not an ideal endpoint for these indolent neoplasms that recur within the first 3 years. During the clinical course of PC, patients experience a progressive increase in calcemia and PTH, and multivariate analysis and risk stratification showed that serum calcium >15 mg/dL at PC diagnosis was negatively associated with RFS (HR = 2.6; 95% CI: 0.91 to 7.6; $P = .0079$).[34] In addition, Xue and colleagues[35] identified that elevated serum calcium (odds ratio [OR] = 7.27; 95% CI: 1.61 to 32.81; $P = .01$) and PTH levels (OR = 1.001; 95% CI: 1.00 to 1.00, $P = .04$) are risk factors for death in patients with PC. The German report by Machens found that a PTH level >700 pg/mL at PC diagnosis was associated with poor CSS (AUC = 0.97, $P = .011$) and, therefore, suggested that suspected or confirmed PCs with PTH >700 should be referred to specialized oncology centers for resolution and follow-up.[36]

Tumor size. The limitations on tumor size as a prognostic factor in PC are due not only to the rarity of this neoplasm but also to deficits with national and international cancer information registry systems. For example, before 1988, tumor size and nodal status were not routinely recorded in North American registry databases, such as SEER. Despite this, in the last 7 years and with the progressive improvement of cancer registry systems, it has been possible to analyze survival according to PC tumor size. In their NCDB study, Asare and colleagues[5] showed that patients with PC tumors >40 mm had an increased risk of death (HR = 1.91; 95% CI, 1.35 to 2.69; $P = .0002$). In addition, adjusting the analysis for nodal status, sex, age at diagnosis, and extent of surgical resection, each centimeter increase in tumor size was associated with a 2% increased risk of death (HR = 1.02, 95% CI: 1.01 to 1.02; $P < .0001$). In univariate and multivariate survival analyses of 520 patients with PC from the SEER dataset, Lo and colleagues[4] detected that tumor size greater than 30 mm (HR = 5.6; 95% CI, 1.5 to 21.2; $P = .011$) was associated with worse DSS. In 2019, Asare and colleagues[8] analyzed the effect of metastasis on survival in a dataset from a tertiary referral cancer hospital. Using recursive partitioning analysis, they showed that primary tumor size greater than 32 mm was the only significant predictor of the development of distant metastasis (HR = 3.51; 95% CI, 1.04 to 11.91; $P = .04$).

Subsequently, in 2022, four studies identified a negative correlation between tumor size and survival in PC. Sun and colleagues[37] analyzed OS and CSS in 209 patients in SEER with confirmed primary PC T1–T2N0M0, which showed that tumor size ≥40 mm was associated with worse CSS (HR = 13.06; 95% CI, 3.75 to 45.51; $P < .001$). On the multivariate analysis based on thyroid invasion, the T2 AJCC TNM 8th Edition, was not an independent risk factor for survival ($P > .05$). In their analysis of CSS in 604 patients with PC, Quian and colleagues[27] showed that tumor size >35 mm (HR = 4.22; 95% CI, 1.67 to 10.68; $P < .002$) was significantly associated with CSS, increasing the risk of cancer-specific death. Ullah and colleagues[28] performed a multivariate survival analysis of 609 patients with PC and showed that tumor size >40 mm was an independent risk factor for mortality ($P < .001$). Finally, a multivariate analysis of 342 patients with PC by Tao and colleagues[29] showed that tumor size >41 mm (HR = 2.18; 95% CI, 1.25 to 3.81; $P = .006$) was an independent variable for OS.

Another notable study, by Wei and colleagues,[38] analyzed 31 reoperations on patients with recurrent or persistent PC and evaluated 5-year OS and DFS. This showed that patients with a compromised upper aerodigestive tract had a 7.6-times increase the risk of mortality (HR = 7.606; $P = .011$) and 5.5-times increase the risk of developing distant metastases (HR = 5.466; $P = .006$).

In conclusion, tumor size alone is a relevant factor to include in a PC staging system, and optimizing data collection on PC in large databases for further analysis in a collaborative and multicentric way is imperative.

Angioinvasion. Angioinvasion is reported in 70% to 90% of PC cases and is considered the most relevant histopathological criterion for malignant diagnosis in parathyroid tumors.[11,39] Historically, angioinvasion has been recognized as a significant and independent predictor of recurrence and death in PC, and it has been included by some authors in their staging systems.[16,22,35,40] In the most recent study, the vascular invasion was one of the most potent independent risk factors for local and distant progression in the multivariate analysis (HR = 3.1; 95% CI, 1.1 to 9.1; $P = .035$). In this study, angioinvasion, age >65 years and serum calcium >15 mg/dL are independent factors negatively associated with relapse-free survival after initial resection of PC.[34]

It is crucial to consider the under-registration of angioinvasion in PC in interpreting these findings. For example, Talat and Schulte conducted an extensive literature review and found that information on angioinvasion was available in only 217 of 1,036 (21%) reported PC cases, which makes it difficult to perform predictive analyses.[16]

Lymph node status. It is known that the reporting of incidence of lymph-node-metastatic disease is variable, ranging between 7% and 32% when such information is available.[1,5,33,41,42] Because the nodal status is unknown in 67% to 75% of cases in the large registry PC databases,[5,29] this prevents correlating this information in multivariate survival analyses. Therefore, its prognostic value is controversial.

The seminal study by Talat and Schulte in 2010 reported that, in the univariate analysis, high-risk patients with PC (vascular invasion, lymph nodes, or distant metastasis) had a 3.5-times higher risk of cancer recurrence and a 4.9-times higher risk of death. This has not been replicated due to the lack of clinical or histopathological nodal status data at the time of PC diagnosis.[16] Hsu and colleagues did not detect, in a multivariate analysis, a specific association between lymph node metastasis and DSS, except for in PCs ≥30 mm (HR = 5.35; 95% CI, 1.5 to 19.5; $P = .01$). Specifically, lymph node metastasis was 7.5 times more likely in patients with PC with tumors ≥30 mm compared with tumors <30 mm (21% vs 2.8%; $P = .02$). Therefore, the use of clinically negative prophylactic central neck dissection might be recommended in tumors ≥30 mm.[33]

Distant metastasis. At diagnosis, fewer than 4% of patients have distant metastases.[16,43] The presence of distant metastases has been consistently found to be a strong prognostic factor in PC for increased risk of death and of poor OS and CSS.

In the SEER study of 520 patients with PC, Lo and colleagues[4] established, in univariate and multivariate analyses, that presence of metastatic disease was associated with worse CSS (HR = 111.4; 95% CI, 20.6 to 601.8; $P < .0001$). Asare and colleagues[5] showed that the 5-year OS of patients with PC who developed distant metastases in the first 5 years was 16% (95% CI, 3% to 91%) compared with 87% (95% CI, 77% to 97%) for those without distant metastases. Furthermore, their study highlighted the fact that patients with bone metastases had an average time to death of 28 months compared with average time to death of 38 months in patients with lung metastases. Therefore, the presence of metastases at the time of diagnosis should be included in a PC staging system.

In addition, distant metastases are an important prognostic factor during the clinical follow-up of PC, because 50% of patients with PC will have local and distant recurrence during clinical follow-up, usually between the second and third year after the first surgical intervention.[16,34,44] Eventually, approximately 25% to 38% of patients will develop distant metastases alone during clinical follow-up.[16,44] The most frequently reported locations of distant disease are the lung (40%) and liver (10%); less frequently, metastases are detected in bone, pleura, brain, pericardium, and pancreas.[14,16]

The most recent reports on PC recurrence with distant metastases showed a 5-year OS of 34%.[38] Tsai and colleagues[45] established in multivariate analyses that bone metastases (HR = 4.83; 95% CI, 1.16 to 20.2; P = .03) and disease-free interval of <1 year (HR = 5.92, 95% CI, 1.85 to 18.99; P = .003) were associated with increased risk of mortality.

Therefore, distant metastases are not only a critical prognostic factor at the time of PC diagnosis but also predict poor survival outcomes when detected during clinical follow-up of all patients with PC.

Microenviromental and tumoral biomarkers

The tumor microenvironment strongly influences the clinical outcomes for patients with PC. Most reports of tumor biomarkers are from original studies and do not come from large databases, because genetic characteristics and molecular mechanisms are usually not recorded in these datasets.

Parafibromin. The *CDC73* mutation has been detected in 15% to 25% of sporadic PCs and in approximately 77% of patients with invasion or metastasis at diagnosis or during clinical follow-up.[46–48] Previous reports attempting to correlate loss of parafibromin staining or *CDC73* mutation with recurrence or death failed to achieve statistical significance due to sample size limitations.[48–52] In the study analyzing 53 patients with PC by Hu and colleagues,[31] negative parafibromin staining was related to recurrence/metastasis (HR = 4.13; 95% CI, 1.73 to 9.87; P = .001). In a meta-analysis of nine studies to estimate the prognostic role of parafibromin in patients with PC,[25] which included 193 well-documented PC cases, absence of parafibromin was a risk factor for recurrence/metastasis (HR = 2.73; 95% CI, 1.43 to 5.21; P = .002) and death (HR = 2.54; 95% CI, 1.35 to 4.76; P = .004). In contrast, *CDC73* mutation was not statistically correlated with DFS or OS; however, age ≥50 years was significantly associated with shorter OS (HR = 2.37; 95% CI, 1.33 to 4.24; P = .004).[25]

In general, despite the inconsistency of results between *CDC73* mutational status and parafibromin staining, parafibromin staining appears to be an easily reproducible, standardized, and promising prognostic factor of survival and relapse in PC.

Intratumoral lymphocytes. Recently, Hu and colleagues[53] studied the intratumoral density of immunocytes and its effect on DFS and OS in 51 patients with PC. Survival analysis showed that the risk factors associated with recurrence/metastasis were low density of CD3+ (P = .017), CD8+ (P = .019), and CD45+ cells (P = .047); a high density of CD163+ cells (P = .003); and a high Ki-67 index (P = .004). The multivariate analysis showed that CD163+ cell density (HR = 16.19; 95% CI, 1.99 to 131.66; P = .009) and CD8+ cell density (HR = 0.13; 95% CI, 0.02 to 0.76; P = .024) were independent factors associated with PC relapse. Kaplan–Meier analysis revealed that high CD8+ cell density correlated with longer OS (P = .047).

Predictive nomogram for survival

Risk assessment models for several cancers are increasingly being published and are often used in clinical practice.[20] They have even been incorporated into the 8th Edition of the AJCC Staging Manual due to their clinical utility while maintaining rigorous and validated evaluation criteria.[24] Although age, gender, metastatic disease, and various biomarkers have been associated with survival in PC (**Fig. 1**; see **Table 3**), each of these factors requires validation in a large international cohort of prospectively collected data. Moreover, so far these factors have not been integrated into an individual survival prediction system.

Tao and colleagues[29] created a predictive nomogram of OS and CSS in PC using 342 PC cases from SEER. Fifty-nine PC cases from a Single Chinese Center Data were used for validation. Based on multivariate analysis, age >66 years (HR = 3.26; 95% CI, 1.87 to 5.69; $P < .001$); tumor size >41 mm (HR = 2.18; 95% CI, 1.25 to 3.81; $P = .006$); and lymph node status positive (HR = 6.68; 95% CI, 2.32 to 19.24; $P < .001$) were independent predictors of OS. In addition, tumor size >41 mm was an independent predictor for CSS (HR = 3.66; 95% CI, 1.57 to 8.54; $P = .003$). These results created a nomogram to predict 3-year, 5-year, and 8-year OS and CSS. In the validation set, the nomogram performed best at predicting 5-year OS (AUC of ROC curves of 0.90) and at predicting 8-year CSS (AUC of ROC curves of 0.94). Although the absolute calibration errors of the nomogram are not established, and the laboratory values (calcium and PTH levels) and some critical histopathological aspects were not included (because they did not have the data for the analysis), this still represents an important initial contribution toward risk staging in PC. Larger cohorts are needed to validate this novel survival prediction approach.

Adjuvant therapy for parathyroid carcinoma

Currently, the surgical resection of the primary tumor with R0 margin is the standard of care for PC, as there is no new evidence that other therapies, such as radiotherapy and chemotherapy, are effective in curing PC or in controlling progression.[10,12,54–56]

Adjuvant external beam radiotherapy. The role of adjuvant EBRT remains controversial for PC. In their 2015 NCDB study, Asare and colleagues[5] reported that only 7% of

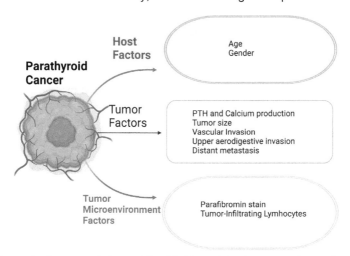

Fig. 1. Schematic of prognostic factors identified in multivariate regression analyses in PC, as reported in the last 7 years in the literature. (*Created with* BioRender.com.)

patients with PCs received RT, and it was not associated with a survival benefit compared with patients who did not receive RT (HR = 1.24; 95% CI, 0.75 to 2.05; P = .4). The HR for RT on OS was 1.4 (95% CI, 0.6 to 3.1; P = .42).

Christakis and colleagues[57] reported on a subgroup of eight patients with PC who had 12.5 years of clinical follow-up at a tertiary referral cancer hospital. These patients received postoperative locoregional RT due to recurrent disease, locally advanced disease, positive margins, and angioinvasion. Of this subgroup, only one patient developed distant metastasis but not until 14 years after the first surgical intervention, and no patient had died as of the last follow-up. In their 2018 SEER study, Lo and colleagues[4] found no significant association between EBRT (9% of patients) and CSS; therefore, the 2016 American Association of Endocrine Surgeons (AAES) guidelines do not recommend routine postoperative EBRT, but it is an option in palliative management.

In their NCDB study of 885 patients with PC by Limberg and colleagues,[58] unadjusted, and multivariate analyses determined that addition of EBRT did not improve OS in the 126 patients who received it (HR = 1.3; 95% CI, 0.9 to 2.0; P = .170 and HR = 1.3; 95% CI, 0.8 to 2.1; P = .320, respectively). Notably, the patient cohort that received EBRT included high-risk patients with locally advanced disease, nodal metastasis, and residual disease. Qian and colleagues[27] also showed that use of RT in the SEER patient dataset of patients with PC did not produce a survival benefit (survival analysis, P = .2; Cox regression analysis, P = .24), and, therefore, RT could not improve CSS. Consensus is that adjuvant RT should be reserved for high-risk patients to control progression, although it does not affect OS.[56,57]

Large datasets (SEER and NCDB) report limited use of ERBT (7% to 16%) and focus on OS versus event-free survival or RFS, which are frequent in PC. The effect of EBRT needs to be investigated in a multi-institutional, long-term standardized study to refine clinical recommendations for its use.

Chemotherapy. Chemotherapy regimens are not standardized for PC, and our knowledge of clinical outcomes is almost entirely from case studies in patients with recurrent and metastatic PC. Monotherapies with dacarbazine or combined with fluorouracil and cyclophosphamide or methotrexate, doxorubicin, and lomustine have been reported.[55,59,60]

Targeted therapies. Recurrence is common in PC, and salvage surgery with medical treatment to control hypercalcemia is recommended palliative care. There is a clinical need for effective and long-acting treatments to control tumor progression and hormonal imbalance due to hypercalcemia.

Efficacy of some targeted therapies in metastatic PC has been reported.[61,62] Sorafenib, a tyrosine kinase inhibitor that inhibits VEGFR-2, VEGFR-3, PDGFR-β, BRAF, FGF receptor 1, RET, and c-kit, angiogenesis receptors described in PC tumorigenesis, was administered to two patients. Both patients presented normalized calcium levels within 9 months of sorafenib use as well as smaller pulmonary lesions upon imaging follow-up.[61,62] Based on these reports, Rozhinskaya and colleagues[63] treated a 27-year-old patient with lung metastases with sorafenib 400 mg twice daily. At publication, the patient had completed 22 months of follow-up and had a normalized biochemical response and a partial regression visualized on DW-MRI that correlated with the anti-angiogenic function of sorafenib. In another study, two patients who developed distant metastases during post-first-surgery follow-up received sorafenib (400 mg, twice daily). One patient progressed during treatment and was then treated with everolimus.[64] These reports are promising and suggest that sorafenib can reduce tumor burden and control serum calcium, which is ultimately the cause of death. Additional studies are warranted to confirm the effects of sorafenib to manage the symptoms of hypercalcemia and to perhaps control long-term disease progression.

Immunotherapy. Tumor response to ICPIs correlates with elevated TMB, >10 mut/Mb, and with an immunogenic tumor microenvironment.[65–67] In several advanced cancers such as melanoma, small-cell lung cancer, and kidney cancer, PD-L1 expression is a biomarker predicting response to anti-PD-L1 or PD-1 treatment.[67] To evaluate whether some patients with PC may benefit from anti-PD-1 or anti-PD-L1 therapy, PD-L1 expression was measured in 18 patients. Four patients had tumors that were PD-L1 positive.[68] Similarly, in another cohort that measured PD-L1 expression and the presence of tumor-infiltrating lymphocytes of 17 patients with PC, four patients were identified with an H-score $\geq$1, and it is hypothesized that these patients may have a positive response to anti-PDI1 therapy.[69,70]

Genomic sequencing of a cohort of PCs identified an association between *CDC73* mutation and high TMB (>20 mut/Mb).[71] Moreover, one patient with an estimated TMB of 5.4 mut/Mb was treated with nivolumab, an anti-PD1 antibody. There was no response after 14 weeks of treatment, and immunohistochemistry confirmed the tumor was PD-L1 negative.[71]

Le and colleagues[72] showed that patients with solid tumors with a deficiency in MSH2, MSH6, PMS2, or MLH1 also had a favorable structural response to PD-1 blockade. This prompted use of Pembrolizumab to treat of a patient with PC with genetically confirmed mismatch repair deficiency (MSH2 and MSH6) who developed pulmonary metastases with hypercalcemia after the first surgical intervention. Pembrolizumab 200 mg was administered every 3 weeks. After the second dose, the patient's PTH and serum calcium levels normalized; however, the fifth and final cycle of Pembrolizumab was discontinued due to colitis and grade 3 to 4 diarrhea. The patient maintained normal biochemistry and clinical presentation through completion of the report.[73]

Genome Profiling and Personalized Cancer Care

Considering the scarcity of targeted drugs to treat PC, and the virtual impossibility of sufficiently large, randomized trials in patients with this rare neoplasm, repurposing of effective targeted therapies to treat patients with PC is a critically important opportunity to advance clinical care (**Table 4**). This approach is increasingly accessible using NGS analyses.

NGS of PCs has identified several candidate driver genes of disease, including *CDC73, CCND1, PRUNE2, PIK3CA, HMT2D, ADCK1, mTOR, THRAP3,* and *CDKN2C.*[74–76] Indeed, mutations in the *TP53* or *PI3K* pathways have been reported in 10% to 30% of genomic sequencing in PC.[74,77] Some of these genes encode proteins for which inhibitor drugs are available and used in other cancer types.[78] In 2019, investigators at MD Anderson Cancer Center performed NGS on tumors from 11 patients with metastatic or recurrent PC.[77] Six tumors had actionable mutations in *ATM, PIK3, TSC1,* or *NF1* that were anticipated to make the tumors sensitive to TOR/PIK3 inhibitors. One patient with a tumor harboring TSC1 mutation was treated with the mTOR inhibitor everolimus to control calcium levels before surgical metastasectomy.[77] Another patient presented with PC with *KDM5C* mutation, which predicted sensitivity to anti-angiogenic drugs.[79] This patient was treated with sorafenib until their serum parameters rose again, and then the patient was switched to another potent angiogenic agent, lenvatinib, which biochemically and structurally stabilized the patient.[77]

Table 4
Summary of potential targeted therapies for specific actionable genetic alterations in parathyroid carcinoma

Mutated Gene	Frequency Reported	Mutation-Specific Treatment[a]
ROS1	26%	Entrectinib and crizotinib
PI3K/AKT/mTOR pathway (ATM, PIK3CA, TSC1, NF1, PTEN, AKT1, mTOR)	35% to 60%	Olaparib, Umbralisib, Duvelisib, Idelalisib, Copanlisib, Alpelisib, Temsirolimus, and Everolimus
ERBB2	5%	Afatinib, Lapatinib, Neratinib, Tucatinib, Trastuzumab, Pertuzumab, and Margetuximab
NTRK1	5%	Larotrectinib and Entrectinib
IDH1	5%	Ivosidenib and Enasidenib
FGFR3	5%	Erdafitinib, Lenvatinib, Pemigatinib, and Infigratinib
ATM	<5%	Olaparib

[a] Approved By National Comprehensive Cancer Network guidelines or FDA for use in solid tumors no-PC.

A similar study by Kang and colleagues[71] identified potentially actionable genomic alterations in 11 of 16 patients with PC. The most frequent mutated genes were *PTEN*, *NF1*, *TSC2*, *KDR*, and *PIK3CA*. The index case showed a KDR T778 K mutation, and the patient was treated with 60 mg/d Cabozantinib, a tyrosine kinase inhibitor with action on VEGFR-2. The patient presented with progressively decreasing PTH levels and a decrease in mediastinal structural damage; unfortunately, therapy was discontinued because of drug-related toxicities. The patient then received a different tyrosine kinase inhibitor, Regorafenib, which resulted in a positive clinical response and was well tolerated.[71]

Cui and colleagues[80] performed a 560-gene panel in 19 PCs, which identified at least one potentially actionable mutation in nine tumors: *ROS1, PTEN, TSC1, PIK3CA, AKT1, mTOR, ERBB2, NTRK1, IDH1*, and *FGFR3*. As in other studies, genes in the PI3K/AKT/mTOR pathway were the most frequently mutated (seven of the nine patients).

Future molecular and genetic characterization of PCs could uncover strategies for personalized adjuvant therapies in advanced or high-risk PC. Genomic profiling should be considered in patients with PC with loss of parafibromin to potentially diagnose *CDC73* mutation or MEN1 syndrome. It should also be considered in all patients with PC who do not achieve remission after the first surgical intervention. Moreover, PCs considered at high risk of recurrence, distant metastases, and death (>40 years, male, high-serum calcium and PTH, tumor size >30 mm, vascular invasion, parafibromin negative, low CD8 cell density, high CD163 cell density, distant or bone metastasis, and early development of metastasis) should always be genetically profiled to identify potential therapeutic interventions. Continued genomic sequencing may also eventually uncover additional pathways involved in parathyroid tumorigenesis, possibly promoting the development of novel drugs.

SUMMARY

The staging systems proposed to date for PC have not been adequately validated. Recent multivariate analyses have been carried out in large national and international databases to search for prognostic factors for survival and relapse in PC. Advanced age, male gender, high PTH and calcium levels at diagnosis, tumor size >30 mm, angioinvasion, presence of distant metastases, and specific tumor microenvironmental factors, such as parafibromin staining and tumor-infiltrating lymphocytes, have been strongly correlated with decreased OS and CSS, and with increased risk of local and distant recurrence. Because of their prognostic significance, these host and tumor factors should be included in any PC staging system. However, there is a need to promote collaborative PC registry plans to collate data on the above prognostic factors as well as new ways in a standardized global registry. Such a resource could be used to stratify patients with PC and identify those at high risk for relapse and death who may benefit from strict surveillance or adjuvant therapeutic care.

PC is an indolent cancer with a high recurrence rate 3 to 5 years after the first surgical intervention. Progression can remain dormant for decades until patients present with distant metastases. Such heterogeneity and neoplastic latency make OS an ambitious endpoint to achieve, and pursuing OS contradicts the actual needs of patients with this endocrine neoplasm. More relevant endpoints focus on achieving normal blood biochemistry to improve quality of life and intervening to lengthen recurrence/metastasis event-related-free survival. Surgery remains the standard treatment because traditional therapies, such as EBRT and chemotherapy, do not benefit patients with advanced unresectable or metastatic PC. Thanks to advances in targeted and immune-based drugs, new options are emerging for patients with PC. Genomic and phenotypic profiling can continue to inform personalized therapeutic strategies to expand the clinical options available to patients with PC.

CLINICS CARE POINTS

- Currently, there is no reliable prognostic prediction system for parathyroid carcinoma (PC).
- In recent studies of large databases, some prognostic factors were identified by multivariate analysis of survival, including original studies and meta-analyses.
- Advanced age, male sex, high parathyroid hormone and calcium levels at diagnosis, tumor size >30 mm, angioinvasion, presence of distant metastases, and specific tumor microenvironmental factors, such as parafibromin staining and tumor-infiltrating lymphocytes, have been correlated with decreases in OC and CSS and with local and distant recurrence.
- A large multi-center study with a unified protocol is still needed to confirm the findings discussed in this review.
- The AJCC 8th Edition Staging Manual requests prospective registration to create a standardized and validated staging system in PC.
- Although, currently, there are no approved systemic therapies for advanced or metastatic PC, use of multi-kinase inhibitors with anti-angiogenesis effects, guided by the identification of mutations in the mTOR/PI3K pathway, can be considered.
- Recent data on the immune compartment in PC have opened new opportunities for research and immune-based therapies to treat advanced or metastatic PC.
- Genetic profiling can be used to understand tumor biology as well as identify rational drug targets.
- Collaborative multi-institutional and multi-disciplinary teams are needed to develop research protocols and clinical trials and to populate robust databases that will identify druggable mutations and associated targeted drugs to deploy in PC.

DISCLOSURE

The author has nothing to disclose.

REFERENCES

1. Lee PK, Jarosek SL, Virnig BA, et al. Trends in the incidence and treatment of parathyroid cancer in the United States. Cancer 2007;109(9):1736–41.
2. Sadler C, Gow KW, Beierle EA, et al. Parathyroid carcinoma in more than 1,000 patients: A population-level analysis. Surgery 2014;156(6):1622–9, discussion 1629-30.
3. Kong SH, Kim JH, Park MY, et al. Epidemiology and prognosis of parathyroid carcinoma: real-world data using nationwide cohort. J Cancer Res Clin Oncol 2021; 147(10):3091–7.
4. Lo WM, Good ML, Nilubol N, et al. Tumor size and presence of metastatic disease at diagnosis are associated with disease-specific survival in parathyroid carcinoma. Ann Surg Oncol 2018;25(9):2535–40.
5. Asare EA, Sturgeon C, Winchester DJ, et al. Parathyroid carcinoma: an update on treatment outcomes and prognostic factors from the national cancer data base (NCDB). Ann Of Surg Oncol 2015;22(12):3990–5.
6. Bilezikian JP, Khan AA, Potts JT Jr. Third International Workshop on the Management of Asymptomatic Primary H. Guidelines for the management of asymptomatic primary hyperparathyroidism: summary statement from the third international workshop. J Of Clin Endocrinol And Metab 2009;94(2):335–9.
7. Duan K, Mete O. Parathyroid Carcinoma: Diagnosis and Clinical Implications. Turk Patoloji Derg 2015;31(Suppl 1):80–97.
8. Asare EA, Silva-Figueroa A, Hess KR, et al. Risk of Distant Metastasis in Parathyroid Carcinoma and Its Effect on Survival: A Retrospective Review from a High-Volume Center. Ann Of Surg Oncol 2019;26(11):3593–9.
9. Fingeret AL. Contemporary Evaluation and Management of Parathyroid Carcinoma. JCO Oncol Pract 2020. https://doi.org/10.1200/JOP.19.00540. JOP1900540.
10. Silva-Figueroa A, Perrier ND. Diagnosis and Surgical Management of Parathyroid Carcinoma. In: Shifrin AL, Raffaelli M, Randolph GW, et al, editors. Endocrine surgery comprehensive board exam guide. Springer International Publishing; 2021. p. 379–403.
11. Erickson LA, Mete O, Juhlin CC, et al. Overview of the 2022 WHO Classification of Parathyroid Tumors. Endocr Pathol 2022;33(1):64–89.
12. Salcuni AS, Cetani F, Guarnieri V, et al. Parathyroid carcinoma. Best Pract Res Clin Endocrinol Metab 2018;32(6):877–89.
13. Sandelin K, Auer G, Bondeson L, et al. Prognostic factors in parathyroid cancer: a review of 95 cases. World J Surg 1992;16(4):724–31.
14. Shane E. Clinical review 122: Parathyroid carcinoma. J Of Clin Endocrinol And Metab 2001;86(2):485–93.
15. Wiseman SM, Rigual NR, Hicks WL Jr, et al. Parathyroid carcinoma: a multicenter review of clinicopathologic features and treatment outcomes. Ear Nose Throat J 2004;83(7):491–4.
16. Talat N, Schulte KM. Clinical presentation, staging and long-term evolution of parathyroid cancer. Ann Surg Oncol 2010;17(8):2156–74.
17. Harari A, Waring A, Fernandez-Ranvier G, et al. Parathyroid carcinoma: a 43-year outcome and survival analysis. J Of Clin Endocrinol And Metab 2011;96(12): 3679–86.

18. Al-Kurd A, Mekel M, Mazeh H. Parathyroid carcinoma. Surg Oncol 2014;23(2): 107–14.
19. Christakis I, Silva AM, Kwatampora LJ, et al. Oncologic progress for the treatment of parathyroid carcinoma is needed. J Surg Oncol 2016. https://doi.org/10.1002/jso.24407.
20. Amin MB, Greene FL, Edge SB, et al. The Eighth Edition AJCC Cancer Staging Manual: Continuing to build a bridge from a population-based to a more "personalized" approach to cancer staging. CA Cancer J Clin 2017;67(2):93–9.
21. Shaha AR, Shah JP. Parathyroid carcinoma: a diagnostic and therapeutic challenge. Cancer 1999;86(3):378–80.
22. Schulte KM, Gill AJ, Barczynski M, et al. Classification of parathyroid cancer. Ann Surg Oncol 2012;19(8):2620–8.
23. Long K, Sippel R. Current and future treatments for parathyroid carcinoma. Int J Endocr Oncol 2018. https://doi.org/10.2217/ije-2017-0011.
24. Amin MB, Edge SB, Green FL, et al. AJCC cancer staging manual. 8th edition. Cham: Springer; 2017.
25. Zhu R, Wang Z, Hu Y. Prognostic role of parafibromin staining and CDC73 mutation in patients with parathyroid carcinoma: A systematic review and meta-analysis based on individual patient data. Clin Endocrinol 2020;92(4):295–302.
26. Leonard-Murali S, Ivanics T, Kwon DS, et al. Local resection versus radical surgery for parathyroid carcinoma: a national cancer database analysis. Eur J Of Surg Oncol 2021;47(11):2768–73.
27. Qian B, Qian Y, Hu L, et al. Prognostic Analysis for Patients With Parathyroid Carcinoma: A Population-Based Study. Front Neurosci 2022;16:784599.
28. Ullah A, Khan J, Waheed A, et al. Parathyroid carcinoma: incidence, survival analysis, and management: a study from the seer database and insights into future therapeutic perspectives. Cancers (Basel) 2022;14(6). https://doi.org/10.3390/cancers14061426.
29. Tao M, Luo S, Wang X, et al. A Nomogram Predicting the Overall Survival and Cancer-Specific Survival in Patients with Parathyroid Cancer: A Retrospective Study. Front Endocrinol 2022;13:850457.
30. Dottorini L, Turati L, Mattei L, et al. Definition and assessment of frailty in older patients: the surgical, anaesthesiological and oncological perspective. Ecancermedicalscience 2020;14:1105.
31. Hu Y, Bi Y, Cui M, et al. The influence of surgical extent and parafibromin staining on the outcome of parathyroid carcinoma: 20-year experience from a single institute. Endocr Pract 2019;25(7):634–41.
32. Wang P, Xue S, Wang S, et al. Clinical characteristics and treatment outcomes of parathyroid carcinoma: A retrospective review of 234 cases. Oncol Lett 2017; 14(6):7276–82.
33. Hsu KT, Sippel RS, Chen H, et al. Is central lymph node dissection necessary for parathyroid carcinoma? Surgery 2014;156(6):1336–41, discussion 1341.
34. Silva-Figueroa AM, Hess KR, Williams MD, et al. Prognostic scoring system to risk stratify parathyroid carcinoma. J Am Coll Surg 2017. https://doi.org/10.1016/j.jamcollsurg.2017.01.060.
35. Xue S, Chen H, Lv C, et al. Preoperative diagnosis and prognosis in 40 Parathyroid Carcinoma Patients. Clin Endocrinol 2016. https://doi.org/10.1111/cen.13055.
36. Machens A, Lorenz K, Dralle H. Parathyroid hormone levels predict long-term outcome after operative management of parathyroid cancer. Horm Metab Res 2017;49(7):485–92.

37. Sun XM, Pang F, Zhuang SM, et al. Tumor size rather than the thyroid invasion affects the prognosis of parathyroid carcinoma without lymph node or distant metastasis. Eur Arch oto-rhino-laryngology 2022. https://doi.org/10.1007/s00405-022-07403-w.

38. Wei B, Zhao T, Shen H, et al. Extended En bloc reoperation for recurrent or persistent parathyroid carcinoma: analysis of 31 cases in a single institute experience. Ann Surg Oncol 2022;29(2):1208–15.

39. DeLellis RA, Larsson C, Arnold A, et al. Tumors of the parathyroid glands. In: R Lloyd R, Osamura G, Kloppel JR, editors. In WHO classification of tumors of endocrine organs. IARC Press; 2017. p. 145–59.

40. Villar-del-Moral J, Jimenez-Garcia A, Salvador-Egea P, et al. Prognostic factors and staging systems in parathyroid cancer: a multicenter cohort study. Surgery 2014;156(5):1132–44.

41. Hundahl SA, Fleming ID, Fremgen AM, et al. Two hundred eighty-six cases of parathyroid carcinoma treated in the U.S. between 1985-1995: a National Cancer Data Base Report. The American College of Surgeons Commission on Cancer and the American Cancer Society. Cancer 1999;86(3):538–44.

42. Schulte KM, Talat N, Miell J, et al. Lymph node involvement and surgical approach in parathyroid cancer. World J Surg 2010;34(11):2611–20.

43. Ferraro V, Sgaramella LI, Di Meo G, et al. Current concepts in parathyroid carcinoma: a single Centre experience. BMC Endocr Disord 2019;19(Suppl 1):46.

44. Sandelin K, Tullgren O, Farnebo LO. Clinical Course of Metastatic Parathyroid Cancer. World J Surg 1994;18(4):594–9.

45. Tsai WH, Zeng YH, Lee CC, et al. Mortality factors in recurrent parathyroid cancer: a pooled analysis. J Bone Miner Metab 2022;40(3):508–17.

46. Gill AJ. Understanding the genetic basis of parathyroid carcinoma. Endocr Pathol 2014;25(1):30–4.

47. Betea D, Potorac I, Beckers A. Parathyroid carcinoma: Challenges in diagnosis and treatment. Ann Endocrinol (Paris) 2015;76(2):169–77.

48. Cetani F, Banti C, Pardi E, et al. CDC73 mutational status and loss of parafibromin in the outcome of parathyroid cancer. Endocr Connect 2013;2(4):186–95.

49. Ryhanen EM, Leijon H, Metso S, et al. A nationwide study on parathyroid carcinoma. Acta Oncol 2017;56(7):991–1003.

50. Guarnieri V, Battista C, Muscarella LA, et al. CDC73 mutations and parafibromin immunohistochemistry in parathyroid tumors: clinical correlations in a single-centre patient cohort. Cell Oncol (Dordr) 2012;35(6):411–22.

51. Wang O, Wang C, Nie M, et al. Novel HRPT2/CDC73 gene mutations and loss of expression of parafibromin in Chinese patients with clinically sporadic parathyroid carcinomas. PloS one 2012;7(9):e45567.

52. Witteveen JE, Hamdy NA, Dekkers OM, et al. Downregulation of CASR expression and global loss of parafibromin staining are strong negative determinants of prognosis in parathyroid carcinoma. Mod Pathol 2011;24(5):688–97.

53. Hu Y, Cui M, Bi Y, et al. Immunocyte density in parathyroid carcinoma is correlated with disease relapse. J endocrinological Invest 2020. https://doi.org/10.1007/s40618-020-01224-6.

54. Cetani F, Pardi E, Marcocci C. Parathyroid Carcinoma. Front Horm Res 2019;51:63–76.

55. Perrier ND, Arnold A, Costa-Guda J, et al. Hereditary endocrine tumours: current state-of-the-art and research opportunities: new and future perspectives for parathyroid carcinoma. Endocr Relat Cancer 2020;27(8):T53–63.

56. Sawhney S, Vaish R, Jain S, et al. Parathyroid carcinoma: a review. Indian J Surg Oncol 2022;13(1):133–42.

57. Christakis I, Silva AM, Williams MD, et al. Postoperative local-regional radiation therapy in the treatment of parathyroid carcinoma: The MD Anderson experience of 35 years. Pract Radiat Oncol 2017;7(6):e463–70.

58. Limberg J, Stefanova D, Ullmann TM, et al. The use and benefit of adjuvant radiotherapy in parathyroid carcinoma: a national cancer database analysis. Ann Surg Oncol 2020. https://doi.org/10.1245/s10434-020-08825-8.

59. Rodrigo JP, Hernandez-Prera JC, Randolph GW, et al. Parathyroid cancer: An update. Cancer Treat Rev 2020;86:102012.

60. Machado NN, Wilhelm SM. Parathyroid Cancer: A Review. Cancers (Basel) 2019; 11(11). https://doi.org/10.3390/cancers11111676.

61. Lerario A, Martin R, Oliveira A, et al. Sorafenib treatment improves refractory hypercalcemia in a patient with metastatic parathyroid carcinoma: a case report. Endocr Soc Poster presented at: 2014; 2014; Chicago. Available at: https://endo.confex.com/endo/2014endo/webprogram/Paper16604.html. Accessed July 15, 2022.

62. Busaidy N, Cabanillas ME, Dadu R, et al. Metastatic parathyroid carcinoma and hypercalcemia responds to treatment with sorafenib. Endocr Soc Poster presented at: 2014; 2014; Chicago. Available at: https://endo.confex.com/endo/2014endo/webprogram/Paper14952.html. Accessed July 15, 2022.

63. Rozhinskaya L, Pigarova E, Sabanova E, et al. Diagnosis and treatment challenges of parathyroid carcinoma in a 27-year-old woman with multiple lung metastases. Endocrinol Diabetes Metab Case Rep 2017;2017. https://doi.org/10.1530/EDM-16-0113.

64. Akirov A, Asa SL, Larouche V, et al. The clinicopathological spectrum of parathyroid carcinoma. Front Endocrinol 2019;10:731.

65. Anagnostou V, Bardelli A, Chan TA, et al. The status of tumor mutational burden and immunotherapy. Nat Cancer 2022;3(6):652–6.

66. Teng MW, Ngiow SF, Ribas A, et al. Classifying cancers based on T-cell Infiltration and PD-L1. Cancer Res 2015;75(11):2139–45.

67. Doroshow DB, Bhalla S, Beasley MB, et al. PD-L1 as a biomarker of response to immune-checkpoint inhibitors. Nat Rev Clin Oncol 2021;18(6):345–62.

68. Du X, Wang L, Shen B, et al. Clinical significance of Pd-L1 expression in parathyroid cancer. Acta Endocrinol (Buchar) 2016;12(4):383–6.

69. Silva-Figueroa A, Villalobos P, Williams MD, et al. Characterizing parathyroid carcinomas and atypical neoplasms based on the expression of programmed death-ligand 1 expression and the presence of tumor-infiltrating lymphocytes and macrophages. Surgery 2018. https://doi.org/10.1016/j.surg.2018.06.013.

70. Spencer KR, Wang J, Silk AW, et al. Biomarkers for immunotherapy: current developments and challenges. Am Soc Clin Oncol Educ Book 2016;35:e493–503.

71. Kang H, Pettinga D, Schubert AD, et al. Genomic profiling of parathyroid carcinoma reveals genomic alterations suggesting benefit from therapy. Oncologist 2019;24(6):791–7.

72. Le DT, Durham JN, Smith KN, et al. Mismatch repair deficiency predicts response of solid tumors to PD-1 blockade. Science 2017;357(6349):409–13.

73. Park D, Airi R, Sherman M. Microsatellite instability driven metastatic parathyroid carcinoma managed with the anti-PD1 immunotherapy, pembrolizumab. BMJ case Rep 2020;13(9). https://doi.org/10.1136/bcr-2020-235293.

74. Pandya C, Uzilov AV, Bellizzi J, et al. Genomic profiling reveals mutational landscape in parathyroid carcinomas. JCI Insight 2017;2(6):e92061.

75. Kasaian K, Wiseman SM, Thiessen N, et al. Complete genomic landscape of a recurring sporadic parathyroid carcinoma. J Pathol 2013;230(3):249–60.
76. Clarke CN, Katsonis P, Hsu TK, et al. Comprehensive genomic characterization of parathyroid cancer identifies novel candidate driver mutations and core pathways. J Endocr Soc 2019;3(3):544–59.
77. Kutahyalioglu M, Nguyen HT, Kwatampora L, et al. Genetic profiling as a clinical tool in advanced parathyroid carcinoma. J Cancer Res Clin Oncol 2019;145(8): 1977–86.
78. Waarts MR, Stonestrom AJ, Park YC, et al. Targeting mutations in cancer. J Clin Invest 2022;132(8). https://doi.org/10.1172/JCI154943.
79. Hsieh JJ, Chen D, Wang PI, et al. Genomic biomarkers of a randomized trial comparing first-line everolimus and sunitinib in patients with metastatic renal cell carcinoma. Eur Urol 2017;71(3):405–14.
80. Cui M, Hu Y, Bi Y, et al. Preliminary exploration of potential molecular therapeutic targets in recurrent and metastatic parathyroid carcinomas. Int J Cancer 2019; 144(3):525–32.

Parathyroid Cancer
Updates and Postoperative Surveillance Imaging

May Thwin, MBBS, MClinSci, Radu Mihai, MD, PhD, FRCS*

KEYWORDS

• Primary hyperparathyroidism • Parathyroid carcinoma • Parathyroid imaging

KEY POINTS

- Imaging after definitive surgical management of parathyroid carcinoma (PC) remains a poorly defined area, and at present, there are no standard guidelines to direct care, which should be individualized and patient-oriented.
- In patients with biochemical or clinical evidence to suggest disease recurrence, imaging aims to identify the culprit site of disease to direct further surgery.
- There is no established role for "routine surveillance" imaging in those patients with sporadic PC who do not display clinical/biochemical signs of disease recurrence.
- Patients diagnosed with a known syndromic gene mutation should have targeted imaging to screen for associated tumors, such as jaw and uterine tumors in the case of hyperparathyroidism-Jaw tumor syndrome.

PARATHYROID CARCINOMA—FREQUENTLY CONSIDERED, RARELY ENCOUNTERED

Most cases of primary hyperparathyroidism (PHPT) are due to benign pathologic condition represented by parathyroid adenomas (up to 85% of patients with PHPT) and multigland hyperplasia (10%–15% of cases).[1,2] In comparison to parathyroid adenomas, it has been reported that only 0.5% to 5% of patients with PHPT have parathyroid carcinoma (PC). Considering the prevalence of PHPT, it may be extrapolated that this low percentage could translate to a relatively large number of patients with PC. However despite this assumption, the quoted incidence of disease does not seem to match the clinical reality, as the largest series of PC included just few hundred cases managed in the United States during several decades (vide infra).

The rarity of the disease is mirrored by a scarcity of articles on the topic of PC. An analysis of research publications during the last 22 years identified only 3578 articles, with relatively flat volume during the entire period and majority focused on the

Financial support: none.
Endocrine Surgery Unit, Churchill Cancer Centre, Oxford University Hospitals NHS Foundation Trust, Oxford OX3 7LE, United Kingdom
* Corresponding author.
E-mail address: Radu.Mihai@ouh.nhs.uk

differential diagnosis, the mechanisms of gene mutation and local tumor recurrence.[3] In this context, there is no level I-III evidence to advise on the ideal postoperative imaging for patients with PC, and clinical practice remains based predominantly on level V evidence (expert opinions).

First described by Sainton and Millot in 1933, PC remains a rare entity and a challenging diagnosis. Clinical presentation lacks specificity for diagnosis, and at present, there is no definitive laboratory test, which can differentiate preoperatively between benign PHPT and PC. Several summarized points are important for the clinician to recognize in oncologic management.

- There is an equal men/women distribution reported for PC, whereas adenomas occur more frequently in women. Patients with PC are on average younger than patients with benign disease but there is a large overlap of age at presentation. Based on data extracted from the Surveillance, Epidemiology, and End Results (SEER) between 1975 and 2016, PC had a minimally higher incidence in men (52.2%), the majority of cases affected Caucasians (75%), and the mean age at diagnosis was 62 years.[4]
- Presentation with a palpable neck mass is highly suggestive of PC. Some centers have reported that this is found in up to 50% of patients with PC[5] but in the experience of the authors, this is an exceedingly rare encounter. Commonly, clinical signs and symptoms of PC are those of hypercalcemia and overlap with those of patients with benign pathologic condition.[6] Therefore, it is impossible to distinguish between the 2 entities based on clinical features, although patients with PC may have more significant morbidity due to the increased severity of their PHPT and hypercalcemia.[6]
- Biochemical abnormalities are more pronounced in PC, and the suspicion of PC is raised preoperatively when patients present with severe hypercalcemia (>3.5 mmol/L) and very high PTH levels. Machado and colleagues[7] (2019) demonstrated higher frequency of symptomatic hypercalcemia, very high serum PTH concentrations greater than 500 mg/dL, serum calcium greater than 14 mg/dL, and presence of so-called parathyroid crisis, defined as rapid onset of corrected serum calcium greater than 14 mg/dL.[7] Patients with PC can have increased presence of combined bone and kidney disease.
- Normocalcemic presentation does not entirely exclude PC because there is a subset of patients with PC who may remain normocalcemic due to nonfunctioning tumors.[7] There are only about 40 patients documented in the literature with PC without high serum PTH.[5] Patients with nonfunctioning PC are documented as presenting in a later and more advanced stage of disease and may have more pathologically aggressive disease with metastases to distant locations including bone and liver.[7]
- A combination of lymphocyte-to-monocyte ratio less than 4.85 in addition to tumor size greater than 28 mm was considered to have a high probability of PC in a study of 36 PCs and 50 benign PT adenomas.[8]

Fine needle aspiration is not a recommended part of preoperative assessment because it can be difficult to distinguish between normal parathyroid tissue, hyperplasia, adenoma, and carcinoma. There is also a risk of "seeding" disease in the biopsy tract, and biopsy can result in hematoma and inflammation, which can increase the difficulty of subsequent surgery.[7]

Preoperative use of ultrasonographic features to differentiate between PC and benign parathyroid disease has been reported recently by Liu and colleagues.[6]

They identified 21 patients with PC and 64 patients with benign parathyroid disease during a 5-year period. The parameters used for the evaluation of lesions included size, shape, borders, margins, internal content, echotexture, echogenicity, calcifications and depth/width ratio, and color Doppler features (**Table 1**). High probability of PC was defined by several parameters: larger size, higher d/W ratio, irregular shape, indistinct border, noncircumscribed margin, cystic change, heterogenous nature, calcifications, and suspicious lymph nodes. The sensitivity of using US to differentiate carcinoma from benign causes was quoted as 65.2% and the specificity 94.4%, and an accuracy of 87.2%.[6]

No published data currently exists on the differentiation of benign disease and carcinoma based on other modalities of preoperative imaging such as (4d)CT scan imaging or Sestamibi-SPECT.

Intraoperatively, demonstrating a large parathyroid tumor with difficult dissection planes toward the thyroid lobe should raise the suspicion of PC and should lead to an *en bloc* resection of the tumor with ipsilateral thyroid lobectomy. This scenario is not common, and it is not always possible to readily differentiate between malignant and benign cause of PHPT intraoperatively[6]; therefore, it remains more common for the diagnosis of PC to be made only after surgery on analysis of the resected specimen.

The histologic criteria for diagnosis of PC were first described by Schantz and Castleman in 1973 as necrosis, mitotic figures, sheets/lobules of tumor cells interspersed with fibrous bands, capsular invasion, and vascular invasion.[9] Of these, the last 2 are regarded as the most representative of malignancy, and PC is confirmed histologically by the presence of vascular invasion alongside immune-histochemical stains used to confirm parathyroid tissue.

The 2022 WHO classification confirmed that the histologic definition of PC still requires one of the following findings: (1) angioinvasion (vascular invasion) characterized by tumor invading through a vessel wall and associated thrombus, or intravascular tumor cells admixed with thrombus, (2) lymphatic invasion, (3) perineural (intraneural) invasion, (4) local malignant invasion into adjacent anatomic structures, or (5) histologically/cytologically documented metastatic disease. In PCs, the documentation of mitotic activity and Ki-67 labeling index is recommended.[10] Adenomas might share some histologic features of carcinomas but lack definitive features of invasive growth.[5]

Parafibromin staining is highly recommended as an auxiliary method in the diagnosis of PC. In a recent study, the loss of parafibromin expression only occurred in malignant tumors, including all carcinomas with metastases (17/17) and 14 of 36 carcinomas with only local infiltration. All staining results of adenomas (53/53) were positive. Considering invasion as the gold standard of malignancy, the sensitivity of

Feature	Parameters
Shape	Round/oval/irregular
Border	Clear/indistinct
Margin	Circumscribed/non
Content	Solid/cystic
Echogenicity	Hypo/iso/hyperechoic
Echotexture	Homo/heterogenous
Doppler features	Vascularization distribution and degree

Table 1
Ultrasound features suggestive of parathyroid carcinoma

Adapted from Liu J, Zhan WW, Zhou JQ, Zhou W. Role of ultrasound in the differentiation of parathyroid carcinoma and benign parathyroid lesions. Clin Radiol. 2020 Mar;75(3):179-184.

parafibromin staining is 58%, and the specificity is 100%. If the gold standard is changed to metastasis, the sensitivity becomes 100%, and the specificity becomes 84%. By analyzing clinicopathological features with metastasis and parafibromin staining, it is found that local-infiltrative carcinomas with positive staining results have better biological behaviors than carcinomas that lack parafibromin expression.[11]

The most recent AJCC Cancer Staging Manual proposed classifying of PC as T1 localized to the parathyroid gland with limited extension to soft tissue; T2 with direct invasion into the thyroid gland; T3 direct invasion into recurrent laryngeal nerve, esophagus, trachea, skeletal muscle, adjacent lymph nodes, or thymus; and T4 direct invasion into major blood vessel or spine. Regional lymph nodes are staged as N0—no regional lymph node metastasis; N1a—metastases to level VI or VII; and N1b—metastases to levels I, II, III, IV, V, or retropharyngeal nodes. Distant metastases are staged as M0 (no distant metastases) or M1 for those with distant disease.[12]

GENETICS

PC may occur as an isolated nonsyndromic case, as a sporadic nonhereditary mutation, or as part of a hereditary disorder.[5] Although most cases with PHPT are sporadic nonsyndromic, up to 5% may be familial, a result of germline mutations in HPT-susceptibility genes[13] (**Table 2**). The most commonly associated hereditary syndromes are hyperparathyroidism-Jaw tumor syndrome (HPT-JT), multiple endocrine neoplasia types 1 and 2 (MEN 1 and MEN 2). PC can affect more than 20% of patients with HPT-JT, an autosomal dominant condition characterized by cancers of the maxilla and mandible, PHPT and in a small subset of patients, tumors of the uterus, and renal cysts. In most cases, the syndrome is caused by a mutation in the CDC73/HRPT2 gene, encoding the protein parafibromin. Mutations of this gene are also seen in 25% of apparently sporadic cases of PC.[13]

Germline heterozygote inactivating mutations of the CDC73 tumor suppressor gene, with somatic loss of heterozygosity at 1q31.2 locus, account for about 50% to 75% of familial cases; more than 75% of sporadic PCs harbor biallelic somatic inactivation/loss of CDC73. Recurrent mutations of the PRUNE2 gene, a recurrent mutation in the ADCK1 gene, genetic amplification of the CCND1 gene, alterations of the PI3K/AKT/mTOR signaling pathway, and modifications of microRNA expression profile and gene promoter methylation pattern have all been detected in PC (**Table 3**).[14]

Given the association of parathyroid cancer and some familial cancer syndromes, the postoperative follow-up of patients with PC should include genetic analysis, and in those found to be identified with mutations, assessment extended to include imaging to screen for associated tumors—such as jaw tumors and uterine tumors in patients with HPT-JT.[15] Discussion of a scheduled regimen for screening in these patients is outside the scope of this article, however, it is important to note that there are currently no established standards or guidelines.

PROGNOSIS OF PARATHYROID CARCINOMA

Resected PC can be associated with high rate of recurrence, prevention of which depends on complete (R0) resection of the tumor.[6] In the absence of an oncological resection, it is quoted that recurrence rate may be greater than 50%, and most of these recurrences are 2 to 3 years after the initial surgery.[7]

Generally, PC has a good prognosis. Ullah and colleagues in their series of 609 patients with PC from the SEER database found overall 1-year, 3-year, and 5-year survival rates of 96%, 89%, and 83%, respectively. Poor survival was associated with

Table 2
Gene mutations associated with malignant parathyroid disease and other syndromes; the proteins they encode, risk of malignancy, and other features of the syndrome

Gene	Protein	Protein Function	Benign or Malignant Parathyroid	Other Associated Conditions Apart from Parathyroid	Additional Imaging Required
CDC73	Parafibromin	Tumor suppressor	~15% malignant	Maxillary/mandible /uterine tumors, renal cysts	Pelvic US, Renal US, CT/MRI
MEN 1	Menin	Tumor suppressor	<1% malignant	MEN 1: Anterior pituitary/ enteropancreatic/ adrenal/foregut carcinoid tumors	
RET	c-Ret	Oncogene	<1% malignant	MEN 2A: medullary thyroid cancer, phaeochromocytoma	

older age, Caucasian ethnicity, male sex, larger tumor size greater than 4 cm, poorly differentiated disease, and distant metastases.[4]

Based on data from 269 cases of PC from the SEER (1989–2014), it was found that thyroid invasion, sex, race, age, radiation, and surgery were not significantly associated with cancer-specific survival by multivariate analysis. However, tumor size 4 cm or greater was significantly associated with worse cancer-specific survival.[16]

In a separate retrospective analysis of 604 PC patients in the SEER database from 2001 through 2018, age at diagnosis greater than 70 years [hazard ratio (HR): 3.55, 95% CI: 1.07 to 11.78] and tumor size greater than 35 mm (HR 4.22, 95% CI: 1.67–10.68) were associated with worse cancer-specific survival.[17]

Using a training dataset of 342 patients with PC was obtained from the SEER database, and a validation dataset included 59 patients from The First Affiliated Hospital of Zhengzhou University only tumor size and stage were predictive for cancer-specific survival,[18] and the authors established a nomogram that can provide accurate prognostics for patients with PC.

FOLLOW-UP PROTOCOLS AFTER RESECTION OF PARATHYROID CARCINOMA

Biochemical monitoring after surgery for PC is based on regular measurements of PTH level and serum calcium/phosphate at 6 to 12 months intervals. In the first few days/weeks after surgery, patients with PC are more likely to develop hungry bone syndrome because of their initial presentation with severe hypercalcemia and very high PTH[7] but within 3 to 6 months postop, they would be expected to stabilize calcium levels.

Routine follow-up imaging after surgery for PHPT is uncommon.[1] There is no current standard accepted protocol when it comes to routine imaging patients after surgically treated PC. Imaging tests should be considered only in patients whose biochemical tests raise suspicion of persistent or recurrent disease. The utility of postoperative imaging is in cases of persistent/recurrent disease to guide further surgery by helping localize the culprit gland/s or possible metastases. Similar to the tests offered at the initial presentation, patients suspected of recurrent disease based on their biochemistry (ie, rising PTH/calcium levels) are recommended to undergo neck ultrasound or MRI combined with functional studies using Sestamibi-Tc^{99m}-SPECT or F^{18}-choline-

Table 3
Most common gene mutations in sporadic parathyroid carcinoma

Gene	Protein	Protein Function	Frequency in PC
CDC73	Parafibromin	Tumor suppressor	70%–100%
CCND 1	Cyclin D1	Proto-oncogene	29%
EZH2	EXH2	Proto-oncogene	60%
PRUNE2	Prune homolog	Tumor suppressor	18%
AKAP9	A-Kinase anchoring protein 9	Proto-oncogene	17.6%
ZEB1	Zinc finger e-box binding homeobox	Proto-oncogene	17.6%

Adapted from Marini F, Giusti F, Palmini G, Perigli G, Santoro R, Brandi ML. Genetics and Epigenetics of Parathyroid Carcinoma. Front Endocrinol (Lausanne). 2022 Feb 24;13:834362.

PET to help localize disease.[7] The US features suggestive of malignancy described above (see **Table 1**) have not been assessed for the diagnosis of recurrent disease.

It remains to be seen who would benefit from the inclusion of imaging in follow-up after surgery for PC. Certainly, its role in those patients with persistent or recurrent disease has been established. However, what of those without clinical and biochemical evidence of disease? It is reasonable that imaging might play a role in surveillance for patients who never had raised PTH and/or calcium to begin with? Moreover, if so, which mode of imaging should be offered, and how do we measure benefits versus cost/risk to the patient, especially if modes of imaging to be offered aside from ultrasound/MRI may expose the patient to unnecessary radiation? So too the role of surveillance imaging for metastases remains undefined. Clinical nomograms have been proposed but little molecular information exists and more research needs to be done to determine who is at risk for metastatic disease (and/or after resection with distant recurrence) and who should be offered screening or surveillance imaging. The role of PRRT and other radioligand pharmaceuticals needs to be explored further in the coming years.

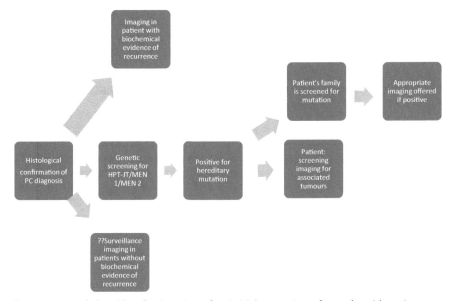

Fig. 1. Proposed algorithm for imaging after initial operation of parathyroid carcinoma.

SUMMARY

Imaging after definitive surgical management of PC remains a poorly defined area, and at present, there are no standard guidelines to direct care, which should be individualized and patient-oriented.

One potential pathway for imaging is proposed in **Fig. 1**. The current role of imaging is largely reserved for patients who demonstrate biochemical or clinical evidence to suggest disease recurrence, and in these patients, imaging is directed at identifying the culprit site of disease to direct further surgery.

There is no established role for "routine" or "surveillance" imaging in those patients with sporadic who do not display signs of disease recurrence.

Patients who are subsequently diagnosed with a known syndromic gene mutation should have targeted imaging to screen for associated tumors, such as jaw and uterine tumors in the case of HPT-JT syndrome.

CLINICS CARE POINTS

- Preoperative suspicion of parathyroid cancer based on severe biochemical abnormalities and suspicious radiological findings should inform the intraoperative decisions about the possible need for ipsilateral thyroid lobectomy.

- Once the histological diagnosis of parathyroid cancer is confirmed, patients should enter a long-term follow-up protocol based predominantly on biochemical screening and imaging initiated if there is any suspicion of disease recurrence.

- Genetic screening should be offered to all patients with a diagnosis of parathyroid carcinoma.

- Developments in imaging techniques and targeted therapy should benefit future patients.

CONFLICT OF INTEREST

None.

DISCLOSURES

The authors have nothing to disclose.

REFERENCES

1. Riley K, Anzai Y. Imaging of Treated Thyroid and Parathyroid Disease. Neuroimaging Clin N Am 2022;32(1):145–57.
2. Yeh MW, Ituarte PH, Zhou HC, et al. Incidence and prevalence of primary hyperparathyroidism in a racially mixed population. J Clin Endocrinol Metab 2013; 98(3):1122–9.
3. Feng C, Tian C, Huang L, et al. A Bibliometric Analysis of the Landscape of Parathyroid Carcinoma Research Based on the PubMed (2000-2021). Front Oncol 2022;12:824201.
4. Ullah A, Khan J, Waheed A, et al. Parathyroid Carcinoma: Incidence, Survival Analysis, and Management: A Study from the SEER Database and Insights into Future Therapeutic Perspectives. Cancers (Basel) 2022;14(6):1426.
5. Cardoso L, Stevenson M, Thakker RV. Molecular genetics of syndromic and nonsyndromic forms of parathyroid carcinoma. Hum Mutat 2017;38(12):1621–48.

6. Liu J, Zhan WW, Zhou JQ, et al. Role of ultrasound in the differentiation of parathyroid carcinoma and benign parathyroid lesions. Clin Radiol 2020;75(3):179–84.
7. Machado NN, Wilhelm SM. Parathyroid Cancer: A Review. Cancers (Basel) 2019;11(11):1676.
8. Ohkuwa K, Sugino K, Katoh R, et al. Preoperative inflammatory markers for predicting parathyroid carcinoma. Endocr Connect 2022;11(7). EC-22-0062.
9. Schantz A, Castleman B. Parathyroid carcinoma. A study of 70 cases. Cancer 1973;31(3):600–5.
10. Erickson LA, Mete O, Juhlin CC, et al. Overview of the 2022 WHO Classification of Parathyroid Tumors. Endocr Pathol 2022;33(1):64–89.
11. Gao Y, Wang P, Lu J, et al. Diagnostic significance of parafibromin expression in parathyroid carcinoma. Hum Pathol 2022;127:28–38.
12. Landry C, Wang T, Asare E. Parathyroid. In: Amin M, editor. AJCC cancer staging manual. 8th edition. Springer International Publishing; 2017. p. 903.
13. Simonds WF. Genetics of Hyperparathyroidism, Including Parathyroid Cancer. Endocrinol Metab Clin North Am 2017 Jun;46(2):405–18.
14. Marini F, Giusti F, Palmini G, et al. Genetics and Epigenetics of Parathyroid Carcinoma. Front Endocrinol (Lausanne) 2022;13:834362.
15. Weaver TD, Shakir MKM, Hoang TD. Hyperparathyroidism-Jaw Tumor Syndrome. Case Rep Oncol 2021;14(1):29–33.
16. Sun XM, Pang F, Zhuang SM, et al. Tumor size rather than the thyroid invasion affects the prognosis of parathyroid carcinoma without lymph node or distant metastasis. Eur Arch Otorhinolaryngol 2022. https://doi.org/10.1007/s00405-022-07403-w. Epub ahead of print. PMID: 35596806.
17. Qian B, Qian Y, Hu L, et al. Prognostic Analysis for Patients With Parathyroid Carcinoma: A Population-Based Study. Front Neurosci 2022;16:784599.
18. Tao M, Luo S, Wang X, et al. A Nomogram Predicting the Overall Survival and Cancer-Specific Survival in Patients with Parathyroid Cancer: A Retrospective Study. Front Endocrinol (Lausanne) 2022;13:850457.

Adrenocortical Carcinoma
Role of Adjuvant and Neoadjuvant Therapy

Lisa Kenney, MD[a],*, Marybeth Hughes, MD[b]

KEYWORDS

- Adrenocortical carcinoma • Mitotane • Adjuvant chemotherapy
- Neoadjuvant chemotherapy

KEY POINTS

- Existing evidence is limited for the use of adjuvant and neoadjuvant chemotherapy in the treatment of adrenocortical carcinoma (ACC).
- The single current US Food and Drug Administration-approved medication for ACC in both treatment and palliation is mitotane.
- The use of adjuvant cytotoxic medications for the treatment of ACC is typically reserved for patients with high risk of recurrence or advanced disease (stage III or greater) and current evidence supports the combination use of etoposide, doxorubicin, cisplatin, and mitotane for these patients.
- Neoadjuvant chemotherapy is used in the treatment of ACC to facilitate complete resection. Much of the rationale for neoadjuvant approach is derived from existing data on adjuvant therapy.
- Surgery remains the only mechanism to cure ACC and should be carefully considered by experienced surgeons in the context of multidisciplinary care.

INTRODUCTION

Following surgical resection of adrenocortical carcinoma (ACC) greater than 50% of patients develop relapse of their disease within 5 years,[1] and a significant number of patients initially present with metastatic disease.[2] Thus, medical therapy is an important component of treatment of this cancer. However, given the rarity of ACC, limited evidence exists for specific regimens of treatment, and there are only a few prospective trials available. Complete surgical resection remains the cornerstone and most important factor in patient outcomes. The single current US Food and Drug Administration approved medication for ACC in both treatment and palliation is mitotane, which acts to inhibit steroidogenesis.[3] However, existing data on mitotane

[a] Department of Surgery, Eastern Virginia Medical School, 825 Fairfax Avenue, Suite 610, Norfolk, VA 23507, USA; [b] Department of Surgery, Division of Surgical Oncology, Eastern Virginia Medical School, 825 Fairfax Avenue, Suite 610, Norfolk, VA 23507, USA
* Corresponding author.
E-mail address: kenneylm@evms.edu

Surg Oncol Clin N Am 32 (2023) 279–287
https://doi.org/10.1016/j.soc.2022.10.005
1055-3207/23/© 2022 Elsevier Inc. All rights reserved.
surgonc.theclinics.com

Table 1
Chemotherapeutic agents that interact with mitotane

Chemotherapeutic Class	Medications
Tyrosine kinase inhibitors	Axitinib[a] Dasatinib Erlotinib Gefitinib Imatinib Nilotinib Lapatinib Sorafenib[a] Sunitinib[a] Vandetanib
mTOR inhibitors	Everolimus[a]
Topoisomerase inhibitors	Etoposide[a]
Vinca alkaloids	Vincristine[a]
Taxols	Docetaxel
Anthracyclines	Doxorubicin[a]

[a] Drugs currently in use or under investigation for use in the treatment of ACC.
Adapted from BRADLOW HL, FUKUSHIMA DK, ZUMOFF B, HELLMAN L, GALLAGHER TF. A Peripheral Action of o,p'-DDD on Steroid Biotransformation, The Journal of Clinical Endocrinology & Metabolism, Volume 23, Issue 9, 1 September 1963, Pages 918–922, https://doi.org/10.1210/jcem-23-9-918.

use for ACC is conflicted and primarily based on retrospective studies. Current standard practice recommendations support combination therapy for mitotane with chemotherapy agents such as etoposide, doxorubicin, and cisplatin, though existing evidence on such treatment is limited.[2,4,5] Current research efforts in this disease process involve determining the molecular characteristics of ACC to find specific targets for therapy, and include strategies for immunotherapy, tyrosine kinase inhibitors, and directed therapies. The need for more comprehensive understanding of this disease limits current options for treatment.

DISCUSSION
Mitotane Therapy

The first clinical application of mitotane, or 2,4'-(dichlorodiphenyl)-2,2-dichloroethane (o,p'-DDD), was discovered in 1949 by Nelson and Woodard when it was observed that the drug caused atrophy of the adrenal cortex in canine models.[6] Initially derived from the pesticide dichlorodiphenyltrichloroethane, this medication has remained a staple of adjuvant therapy for ACC since its application in human patients in 1960,[7] although the full mechanism of action is still being investigated. Although the effect of mitotane varies between species, it is recognized that high levels damage the zona fasciculata and reticularis of the adrenal gland in humans, whereas the zona glomerulosa is spared. On a cellular level, it acts on the mitochondria to affect membranes of the respiratory chain.[8] Studies investigating the effects of mitotane on steroidogenesis show inhibitory effects on the synthesis of 11β-hydroxylase, 3β-hydroxysteroid dehydrogenase, and 18-hydroxylase.[9,10] As an inducer of cytochrome CYP34A, mitotane affects the metabolism of several medications, including other chemotherapeutic agents in use for ACC.[11] **Table 1** lists known therapies for ACC affected by mitotane. Patients who are on mitotane often experience significant side effects including alterations to thyroid and testosterone metabolism, especially at the targeted therapeutic level of 14 to 20 mcg/mL. Patients on mitotane therapy will also typically need long-term glucocorticoid replacement therapy.[12,13]

The 2018 European Society of Endocrinology (ESE) Clinical Practice Guidelines recommend the use of mitotane for patients with ACC, particularly in patients who have at least one feature: (1) stage III disease, (2) R1-surgical resection, or (3) Ki67 greater than 10%. Those without such characteristics should be evaluated on an individual basis for mitotane therapy.[14] Thus, mitotane is supported in patients who are deemed high risk for recurrence. However, questions remained on the appropriate use of mitotane in those deemed low risk.

The first randomized trial on adjuvant mitotane in ACC patients, known as the Adjuvo study, sought to fill the recommendation gap from the ESE Clinical Practice Guidelines on the use of mitotane in ACC patients with low or intermediate risk of recurrence. The inclusion criteria were (1) stage I to III disease, R0 surgery, and Ki-67 less than 10%. They were randomized to mitotane therapy or observation after resection. A total of 91 patients were enrolled with 45 in the mitotane arm and 46 in the observational arm. The results of the study found no difference recurrence free survival (RFS) in this subset of patients, with the hazard ratio (HR) for recurrence was 1.321 (95% CI, 0.55–3.32, $P = .54$) and HR for death 2.171 (95% CI, 0.52–12.12, $P = .29$). Thus, mitotane was not recommended for low to intermediate recurrence risk ACC patients after resection.[15]

A recent meta-analysis on prognostic benefits of adjuvant mitotane after resection of ACC in patients without distant metastasis was performed by Tang *and colleagues* at Sichuan University in Chengdu, China, and included 5 studies (which were all retrospective) reporting on 1249 patients. The meta-analysis found significantly longer RFS (HR = 0.62; 95% CI, 0.42–0.94; $P < .05$) and prolonged overall survival (OS; HR = 0.69; 95% CI, 0.55–0.88, $P < .05$), supporting the use of adjuvant mitotane in ACC. The authors specifically excluded studies, which involved patients with metastatic disease, no prior resection of the tumor, neoadjuvant therapy before surgery, or other chemotherapeutic agents in addition to mitotane. However, adjuvant radiotherapy was allowed as part of the meta-analysis. The patients were not stratified based on stage of disease, resection margins, or Ki67 percentage.[16] Thus, the authors suggest that monotherapy with mitotane is beneficial in the adjuvant setting for patients who show no signs of metastasis.

Adjuvant Chemotherapy, Immunotherapy, and Targeted Therapies

The use of adjuvant cytotoxic medications for the treatment of ACC is still debated and is typically reserved for patients with high risk of recurrence or advanced disease (stage III or greater), as most existing studies have small enrollment sizes and the benefit is not clear. The introduction and use of immunotherapies and targeted therapies, such as use of monoclonal antibodies, checkpoint inhibitors, and tyrosine kinase inhibitors in cancer treatment has been an area of recent interest in the treatment of ACC.[17] Such therapies can be devised by understanding the mechanisms by which cancer cells escape surveillance of the immune system. Thus, several trials involving monoclonal antibodies such as anticytotoxic T cell antigen 4 (anti-CTLA-4), antiprogrammed cell death protein 1 (anti-PD-1), and antiprogrammed cell death protein ligand 1 (anti-PD-L1) against various types of cancer are being studied (Refer to **Table 2**). However, no significant breakthrough for ACC has been discovered thus far for these novel types of treatments.

The first phase 3 clinical trial involving systemic therapy for ACC was published in 2012. Known as the First International Randomized Trial in Locally Advanced and Metastatic Adrenocortical Carcinoma Treatment (FIRM-ACT), it compared the treatment

Table 2
Relevant clinical trials investigating the use of adjuvant chemotherapy, immunotherapy, and targeted therapies in the treatment of ACC, 2012–2022

Reference	Chemotherapy	Number of Patients	Results
Fassnacht et al,[18] 2012	Mitotane plus etoposide, doxorubicin, and cisplatin vs mitotane plus streptozocin	304 with advanced ACC	Higher response rate (23.2% vs 9.2%, $P < .001$) and longer median PFS (5.0 vs 2.1 mo, HR 0.55; 95% CI, 0.43–0.69; $P < .001$) in mitotane plus etoposide, doxorubicin, and cisplatin group. No significant difference in OS
Berruti et al,[20] 2012	Sorafenib (kinase inhibitor) plus metronomic paclitaxel	25 with metastatic ACC	No benefit
Kroiss et al,[21] 2012	Sunitinib (kinase inhibitor)	38 patients with refractory ACC (after treatment with mitotane and cytotoxic chemotherapy)	5 patients experienced stable disease, 24 had progressive disease, and 6 patients died from ACC before the first evaluation; also had some evidence of drug interaction with mitotane
Urup et al,[22] 2013	Cisplatin plus docetaxel	19 with advanced ACC	The response rate was 21% (95% CI: 3%–39%). No patients obtained a complete response, 32% had stable disease, and 37% progressed while on treatment. The median PFS was 3 mo (95% CI: 0.7–5.3 mo)
Naing et al,[23] 2013	Cixutumumab (monoclonal antibody against IGF-1R) plus temsirolimus	20 with metastatic ACC	Stable disease >6 mo (range 6–21 mo) in 42% of participants
O'Sullivan et al,[24] 2014	Axitinib (tyrosine kinase inhibitor)	13 with metastatic ACC (previously treated with at least 1 chemotherapy regimen with or without mitotane)	No benefit

Fassnacht et al,[25] 2015	Linsitinib (inhibitor of IGF-1R)	139 locally advanced or metastatic ACC	No benefit
Le Tourneau et al,[26] 2018	Avelumab (monoclonal antibody against PD-L1)	50 with metastatic ACC (previously treated)	The response rate was 6% (95% CI: 1.3%–16.5%). 42% had stable disease. Median PFS was 2.6 mo (95% CI: 1.4–4.0)
Habra et al,[27] 2019	Pembrolizumab (monoclonal antibody against PD-1 receptor)	16 with ACC (prior treatment failure in last 6 mo), 2 lost to follow-up	The response rate was 14% (95% CI: 2%–43%). At 27 wk, 2 had a partial response, 7 had stable disease, and 5 had progressive disease
Carneiro et al,[28] 2019	Nivolumab (monoclonal antibody against PD-1 receptor)	10 with metastatic ACC (previously treated with platinum-based chemotherapy or mitotane)	Median PFS was 1.8 mo (95% CI, 0.1–4.3). 2 of the 10 participants showed stable disease for 48 and 11 wk
Raj et al,[29] 2020	Pembrolizumab (monoclonal antibody against PD-1 receptor)	39 with advanced ACC	Objective response rate was 23% (95% CI: 11%–39%). Median PFS was 2.1 mo (95% CI: 2.0–10.7)

Adapted from Paragliola RM, Corsello A, Locantore P, Papi G, Pontecorvi A, Corsello SM. Medical Approaches in Adrenocortical Carcinoma. Biomedicines. 2020;8(12):551. Published 2020 Nov 29. https://doi.org/10.3390/biomedicines8120551.

of metastatic ACC with etoposide, doxorubicin, cisplatin, and mitotane (EDP–mitotane group) versus treatment with streptozotocin and mitotane (streptozocin–mitotane group). This was a randomized controlled trial that was conducted in 12 countries at 40 specialized centers and thus had a higher participant enrollment than all prior phase 2 trials combined at the time, with 304 total enrolled patients. The patients in the EDP–mitotane group had a significantly higher response rate than those in the streptozocin–mitotane group (23.2% vs 9.2%, $P < .001$) and longer progression-free survival (PFS; 5.0 vs 2.1 months; HR 0.55 95% CI, 0.43–0.69; $P < .001$). There was no significant between-group difference in OS (OS; 14.8 and 12.0 months, 95% CI, 0.61–1.02; $P = .07$).[18] A retrospective study in Tokyo, Japan, involving 43 patients with metastatic ACC at the National Cancer Center Hospital between 1997 and 2020 showed similar outcomes to the FIRM-ACT trial, with a median PFS of 6.2 months (95% CI: 4.3–10.0) and OS of 15.4 months (95% CI 11.6–not reached).[19] **Table 2** references the relevant clinical trials (2012–2022) involving systemic chemotherapy and immunotherapy in the treatment of ACC.

Neoadjuvant Chemotherapy

Although adjuvant therapy for the treatment of ACC has been a topic of research for decades, the concept of neoadjuvant therapy is a more recent consideration. The current consensus for use of systemic neoadjuvant chemotherapy in ACC is to reduce the burden of disease to facilitate complete resection.[30] Most experts do not recommend neoadjuvant treatment when R0 surgical resection is possible upfront (**Fig. 1** below, treatment algorithm for ACC). Much of the rationale for neoadjuvant approach is derived from existing data on adjuvant therapy. Currently, there is a single retrospective study from MD Anderson Cancer Center evaluating the use of neoadjuvant chemotherapy for patients with borderline resectable ACC (BRACC), defined as tumor or patient characteristics at presentation that argue against immediate surgery because of an unacceptable risk of morbidity/mortality, incomplete resection, or

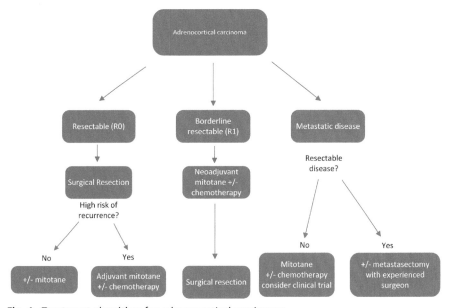

Fig. 1. Treatment algorithm for adrenocortical carcinoma.

recurrence. The study included 53 patients with ACC, 15 (28.3%) of which were considered BRACC and underwent neoadjuvant therapy. Of these 15 patients, 12 (80%) received mitotane and etoposide/cisplatin-based chemotherapy, 2 (13%) received mitotane alone, and 1 (7%) received chemotherapy alone. Median disease-free survival for resected BRACC patients who underwent neoadjuvant therapy was higher than the patients who underwent surgery for initial treatment, at 28.0 months (95% CI 2.9–not attained) versus 13 months (95% CI 5.8–46.9; P = .40). Five-year OS was similar between the groups as well (65% vs 50%, P = .72).[31,32] Neoadjuvant therapy in the setting of borderline resectable disease is appropriate for the facilitation of R0 resection, and prospective randomized trials would further determine the benefit of neoadjuvant chemotherapy for these patients.

Surgery remains the only mechanism to cure ACC and should be carefully considered by experienced surgeons in the context of multidisciplinary care.

SUMMARY

Current evidence regarding the use of adjuvant and neoadjuvant chemotherapy in the treatment of ACC is limited by mostly retrospective studies. The use of mitotane has been long used in the treatment of ACC but consensus only supports its use for adjuvant therapy in cases of high risk of recurrence because it has questionable benefit and has many known side effects and drug interactions. Evidence regarding the use of systemic chemotherapy is limited by small sample sizes, and treatment is reserved for patients with high risk of recurrence or advanced disease (stage III or greater). The FIRM-ACT trial was the first phase 3 trial involving systemic chemotherapy and is the basis for use of etoposide, doxorubicin, cisplatin, and mitotane as combination therapy. Although the use of targeted therapies and immunotherapy for ACC is promising, breakthroughs have not yet been made. Neoadjuvant therapy in ACC is typically not recommended unless R0 resection is not possible upfront, and limited studies show some benefit of neoadjuvant therapy to facilitate complete surgical removal of tumor. Surgical excision is the definitive treatment of ACC.

CLINICS CARE POINTS

- Surgical excision is the cornerstone of ACC treatment.
- Adjuvant mitotane therapy is generally recommended for ACC in the context of high risk of recurrence or for palliation of symptoms.
- Systemic chemotherapy is used for patients with high risk of recurrence or advanced disease (stage III or greater). Current evidence supports the combination use of etoposide, doxorubicin, cisplatin, and mitotane as combination therapy.
- Neoadjuvant chemotherapy is considered to facilitate R0 resection, and no current guidelines exist for specific neoadjuvant therapies.

DISCLOSURE

The authors have nothing to disclose.

REFERENCES

1. Glover AR, Ip JC, Zhao JT, et al. Current management options for recurrent adrenocortical carcinoma. Onco Targets Ther 2013;6:635–43.

2. Bianchini M, Puliani G, Chiefari A, et al. Metabolic and endocrine toxicities of mitotane: a systematic review. Cancers (Basel) 2021;13(19):5001.

3. Assié G, Antoni G, Tissier F, et al. Prognostic parameters of metastatic adrenocortical carcinoma. J Clin Endocrinol Metab 2007;92(1):148–54.

4. Kiseljak-Vassiliades K, Bancos I, Hamrahian A, et al. American association of clinical endocrinology disease state clinical review on the evaluation and management of adrenocortical carcinoma in an adult: a practical approach. Endocr Pract 2020;26(11):1366–83.

5. Postlewait LM, Ethun CG, Tran TB, et al. Outcomes of Adjuvant Mitotane after Resection of Adrenocortical Carcinoma: A 13-Institution Study by the US Adrenocortical Carcinoma Group. J Am Coll Surg 2016;222(4):480–90 [published correction appears in J Am Coll Surg. 2018 Jan;226(1):114].

6. Terzolo M, Fassnacht M, Perotti P, et al. Results of the ADIUVO Study, the First Randomized Trial on Adjuvant Mitotane in Adrenocortical Carcinoma Patients. J Endocr Soc 2021;5(Suppl 1):A166–7. Published 2021 May 3.

7. Nelson AA, Woodard G. Severe adrenal cortical atrophy (cytotoxic) and hepatic damage produced in dogs by feeding 2,2-bis(parachlorophenyl)-1,1-dichloroethane (DDD or TDE). Arch Pathol (Chic) 1949;48(5):387–94.

8. Bergenstal DM, Hertz R, Lipsett MB, et al. Chemotherapy of adrenocortical cancer with o,p'ddd. Ann Intern Med 1960;53(4):672–82.

9. Hescot S, Amazit L, Lhomme M, et al. Identifying mitotane-induced mitochondria-associated membranes dysfunctions: metabolomic and lipidomic approaches. Oncotarget 2017;8(66):109924–40. https://doi.org/10.18632/oncotarget.18968. Published 2017 Jul 4.

10. Bradlow HL, Fukushima DK, Zumoff B, et al. A peripheral action of o,p' -ddd on steroid biotransformation. J Clin Endocrinol Metab 1963;23:918–22.

11. Brown RD, Nicholson WE, Chick WT, et al. Effect of o,p'DDD on human adrenal steroid 11 beta-hydroxylation activity. J Clin Endocrinol Metab 1973;36(4):730–3.

12. Kroiss M, Quinkler M, Lutz WK, et al. Drug interactions with mitotane by induction of CYP3A4 metabolism in the clinical management of adrenocortical carcinoma. Clin Endocrinol (Oxf) 2011;75(5):585–91.

13. Berruti A, Fassnacht M, Libè R, et al. First randomized trial on adjuvant mitotane in adrenocortical carcinoma patients: the adjuvo study. J Clin Oncol 2022; 40(6_suppl):1.

14. Paragliola RM, Torino F, Papi G, et al. Role of mitotane in adrenocortical carcinoma - review and state of the art. Eur Endocrinol 2018;14(2):62–6.

15. Tang Y, Liu Z, Zou Z, et al. Benefits of adjuvant mitotane after resection of adrenocortical carcinoma: a systematic review and meta-analysis. Biomed Res Int 2018;2018:9362108.

16. Fassnacht M, Assie G, Baudin E, et al. Adrenocortical carcinomas and malignant phaeochromocytomas: ESMO-EURACAN clinical practice guidelines for diagnosis, treatment and follow-up. Ann Oncol 2020;31(11):1476–90.

17. Karwacka I, Obołończyk Ł, Kaniuka-Jakubowska S, et al. The Role of Immunotherapy in the Treatment of Adrenocortical Carcinoma. Biomedicines 2021; 9(2):98.

18. Fassnacht M, Terzolo M, Allolio B, et al. Combination chemotherapy in advanced adrenocortical carcinoma. N Engl J Med 2012;366(23):2189–97.

19. Uchihara M, Tanioka M, Kojima Y, et al. Clinical management and outcomes associated with etoposide, doxorubicin, and cisplatin plus mitotane treatment in metastatic adrenocortical carcinoma: a single institute experience. Int J Clin Oncol 2021;26(12):2275–81.

20. Berruti A, Sperone P, Ferrero A, et al. Phase II study of weekly paclitaxel and sorafenib as second/third-line therapy in patients with adrenocortical carcinoma. Eur J Endocrinol 2012;166(3):451–8.

21. Kroiss M, Quinkler M, Johanssen S, et al. Sunitinib in refractory adrenocortical carcinoma: a phase II, single-arm, open-label trial. J Clin Endocrinol Metab 2012;97(10):3495–503.

22. Urup T, Pawlak WZ, Petersen PM, et al. Treatment with docetaxel and cisplatin in advanced adrenocortical carcinoma, a phase II study. Br J Cancer 2013;108(10): 1994–7.

23. Naing A, Lorusso P, Fu S, et al. Insulin growth factor receptor (IGF-1R) antibody cixutumumab combined with the mTOR inhibitor temsirolimus in patients with metastatic adrenocortical carcinoma. Br J Cancer 2013;108(4):826–30.

24. O'Sullivan C, Edgerly M, Velarde M, et al. The VEGF inhibitor axitinib has limited effectiveness as a therapy for adrenocortical cancer. J Clin Endocrinol Metab 2014;99(4):1291–7.

25. Fassnacht M, Berruti A, Baudin E, et al. Linsitinib (OSI-906) versus placebo for patients with locally advanced or metastatic adrenocortical carcinoma: a double-blind, randomised, phase 3 study. Lancet Oncol 2015;16(4):426–35. https://doi.org/10.1016/S1470-2045(15)70081-1.

26. Le Tourneau C, Hoimes C, Zarwan C, et al. Avelumab in patients with previously treated metastatic adrenocortical carcinoma: phase 1b results from the JAVELIN solid tumor trial. J Immunother Cancer 2018;6(1):111.

27. Habra MA, Stephen B, Campbell M, et al. Phase II clinical trial of pembrolizumab efficacy and safety in advanced adrenocortical carcinoma. J Immunother Cancer 2019;7(1):253.

28. Carneiro BA, Konda B, Costa RB, et al. Nivolumab in metastatic adrenocortical carcinoma: results of a phase 2 trial. J Clin Endocrinol Metab 2019;104(12): 6193–200.

29. Raj N, Zheng Y, Kelly V, et al. PD-1 blockade in advanced adrenocortical carcinoma. J Clin Oncol 2020;38(1):71–80.

30. Yip L, Duh QY, Wachtel H, et al. American Association of Endocrine Surgeons Guidelines for Adrenalectomy: Executive Summary. JAMA Surg 2022;157(10): 870–7.

31. Bednarski BK, Habra MA, Phan A, et al. Borderline resectable adrenal cortical carcinoma: a potential role for preoperative chemotherapy. World J Surg 2014; 38(6):1318–27.

32. Paragliola RM, Corsello A, Locantore P, et al. Medical approaches in adrenocortical carcinoma. Biomedicines 2020;8(12):551.

Succinate Dehydrogenase Mutations as Familial Pheochromocytoma Syndromes

Michael S. Lui, MD[a,1], Uriel Clemente-Gutierrez, MD[a,1],
Catherine M. Skefos, MA, MS[b], Nancy D. Perrier, MD[a,*]

KEYWORDS

- Hereditary pheochromocytoma/paraganglioma • Genetic testing • Adrenalectomy
- Metastatic pheochromocytoma/paraganglioma • Preoperative blockade
- Succinate dehydrogenase subunit B (SDHB)

KEY POINTS

- Patients with pheochromocytomas/paragangliomas (PPGLs) frequently have germline mutations and should undergo genetic testing.
- Those with succinate dehydrogenase subunit B (SDHB) mutations have a higher risk of developing metastatic PPGLs and should undergo open surgical resection at experienced, specialized centers.
- Resection of the primary tumor may still increase overall survival and provide symptomatic relief in patients presenting with metastatic PPGLs.
- All PPGLs have malignant potential and requires up to 10 years of surveillance. Those with germline mutations associated with PPGLs or high-risk features for metastatic disease need lifelong surveillance.

INTRODUCTION

Pheochromocytomas and paragangliomas (PPGLs) are rare neuroendocrine tumors with an estimated annual incidence of two to eight cases per 1,000,000 persons.[1] Although both are embryologically of neural crest origin, pheochromocytomas are tumors that specifically arise from the chromaffin cells of the adrenal medulla whereas paragangliomas can arise anywhere along the extra-adrenal sympathetic/parasympathetic paraganglia. PPGLs are classically described as functional tumors associated

[a] Department of Surgical Oncology, Division of Surgical Endocrinology, The University of Texas MD Anderson Cancer Center, 1400 Pressler Street, Unit 1484, Houston, TX 77030, USA; [b] Clinical Cancer Genetics Program, Division of Surgical Endocrinology, The University of Texas MD Anderson Cancer Center, Houston, TX, USA
[1] These authors contributed equally and are co-first authors.
* Corresponding author.
E-mail addresses: Michael.Lui@nyulangone.org (M.S.L.); Uclementeg@gmail.com (U.C.-G.); CBSkefos@mdanderson.org (C.M.S.); nperrier@mdanderson.org (N.D.P.)

Surg Oncol Clin N Am 32 (2023) 289–301
https://doi.org/10.1016/j.soc.2022.10.006

Abbreviations	
18F-FDG PET	Flourine-18 2-fluoro-2-deoxy-D-glucose positron emission tomography
AJCC	American Joint Committee on Cancer
CSDE1	Cold shock domain-containing E1 gene
GIST	Gastrointestinal stroma tumors
FH	Fumarate hydratase
HIF1a	Hypoxia induced factor 1 gene
HNPGL	Head and neck paraganglioma
HSA	High-specific-activity
MAML3	Mastermind-like transcriptional coactivator 3 gene
MAX	Myc-associated factor X gene
MDH2	Malate dehydrogenase 2
MEN2	Multiple endocrine neoplasia type 2
MIBG	Metaiodobenzylguanidine
MTOR	Mechanistic target of rapamycin gene
NF1	Neurofibromatosis type 1 gene
NGS	Next generation sequencing
PGLx	Paraganglioma syndrome type x
PPGL	Pheochromocytoma/Paraganglioma
RCT	Randomized controlled trial
SDHx	Succinate dehydrogenase subunit x
SDHAF2	Succinate dehydrogenase assembly factor 2 gene
SEER	Surveillance, Epidemiology, and End Results
TCGA	The Cancer Genome Atlas
TMEM127	Transmembrane protein 127 gene
VHL	Von Hippel Lindau

with excess catecholamine secretion, but like other neuroendocrine tumors, they may also present as non-functional lesions. Morbidity and mortality associated with PPGL are commonly due to catecholamine excess, local invasion, and/or metastatic disease, which is defined as the presence of PPGL in tissue(s) normally void of chromaffin cells. Over the past decade, there has been a shift away from describing PPGL as "benign" or "malignant" to those with or without the metastatic disease to acknowledge the fact that *all* PPGL have malignant potential. In 2017, the American Joint Committee on Cancer (AJCC) developed a PPGL staging system to be used for all PPGLs to better prognosticate patients.[2]

It was historically believed that hereditary PPGL made up a small portion of PPGL presentations. However, as more PPGL susceptibility genes are identified, it is now believed that up to 40% of PPGL cases are associated with a germline mutation.[3] Depending on the mutation, clinicians can make predictions on tumor behavior as well as become vigilant toward identifying other syndromic manifestations. The following sections will discuss the role and importance of genetic testing for all patients with PPGLs and its implications on preoperative, perioperative, and postoperative management, especially in the setting of succinate dehydrogenase subunit B (SDHB)-associated PPGL.

GENETIC TESTING
Genotype Clustering

Before the twenty-first century, multiple endocrine neoplasia type 2 (MEN2), neurofibromatosis type 1 (NF1), and von Hippel-Lindau (VHL) disease were the primary known syndromes associated with PPGL development.[4] More recently, additional somatic and germline drivers of PPGL growth have been identified. Although the pathologic pathway for some mutations remains elusive, analysis from The Cancer Genome

Atlas network identified three pathways ("clusters") believed to be the drivers for onco-genesis: (1) Cluster 1: pseudohypoxia pathway, (2) Cluster 2: kinase-signaling pathway, and (3) Cluster 3: Wnt signaling pathway.[5] Cluster 1 mutations include *VHL*, *SDHx*,[6] fumarate hydratase (*FH*),[7] malate dehydrogenase 2 (*MDH2*),[8] and hypoxia-inducible factor 2 alpha (*HIF2a*),[9] all of which result in the stabilization of HIF1a, which in turn, upregulates gene transcription stimulating cellular proliferation and angiogenesis.[6] Cluster 2 mutations include *RET*, *NF1*, transmembrane protein 127 (*TMEM127*),[10] and Myc-associated factor X (*MAX*).[11] These mutations cause autonomous activation of the mitogen-activated protein kinase pathway via activation of RAS (*NF1* mutation), mechanistic target of rapamycin (*MTOR*; *TMEM127* mutation), Myc (*MAX* mutation) or the tyrosine kinase transmembrane receptor (*RET* mutation) causing cellular growth and proliferation.[3] Lastly, cluster 3 remains largely unexplored, but is believed to be caused by somatic mutations in mastermind-like transcriptional coactivator 3 (*MAML3*) and cold shock domain-containing E1 gene (*CSDE1*) activating Wnt and Hedgehog signaling to increase angiogenesis and cellular proliferation and survival.[5] Although the identification of PPGL-susceptible mutations can hint at the likely behavior of the PPGL, leveraging our understanding of the pathologic pathway to develop targeted therapeutics for precision medicine remains an area of interest.

Familial Paraganglioma Syndrome

In the early 2000s, it was identified that a succinate dehydrogenase (SDH) germline mutation was associated with an increased risk of developing PPGLs.[12–14] SDH mu-tations make up a significant portion of cluster 1 (pseudohypoxia) mutations. Normally, SDH is a heterotetrameric mitochondrial protein complex that participates in cellular aerobic respiration by transforming succinate into fumarate, ultimately contributing to the electron transport chain. Mutations in this complex will stall oxidative phosphor-ylation causing cells to shift to the inefficient anaerobic cellular respiration pathway. As previously mentioned, these mutations create a pseudohypoxic environment which will stabilize HIF1a, signal the hypoxic pathway, and lead to angiogenesis and cellular proliferation.[6]

Paraganglioma tumor syndrome (also known as SDHx-associated hereditary pheo-chromocyotoma and paraganglioma syndrome) is caused by mutations in any of the genes that contribute to the SDH complex (SDHA, SDHAF2, SDHB, SDHC, SDHD) and is referred to as PGL1-5.[15] PGL1 is the most common variant and is caused by mutations in *SDHD* which encodes the D subunit of the SDH complex. Seventy-five percent of the carriers will develop a tumor by age 40 and are more likely to develop paragangliomas in the head and neck (HNPGL) as opposed to the abdomen or tho-rax.[16,17] While the majority of cases will present with multifocal tumors, metastases are rarely seen in PGL1 patients.[17,18] Only a few families have been diagnosed with a mutation in SDH assembly factor 2 (SDHAF2) and are classified as PGL2. Like those patients with *SDHD* mutation, these patients typically present with multifocal HNPGL and have not been reported to have an increased risk of metastatic disease.[19] The PGL3 syndrome is seen in patients with mutations in *SDHC*, and is characterized by the development of HNPGL, but unlike PGL1 and PGL2, most often presents as a sin-gle carotid body tumor.[18] The reported metastatic potential for those with PGL3 is low.[18] PGL4 is caused by mutations in *SDHB* and is more likely to be associated with thoracoabdominal PPGL. Most clinically relevant is the fact that patients with a *SHDB* mutation have a 30% to 70% risk of developing synchronous or metachronous metastatic disease.[20] Additionally, *SDHB* mutations have been associated with non-PPGL tumors including gastrointestinal stromal tumors (GISTs), papillary thyroid can-cer, and neuroblastoma or renal cell carcinomas.[21] Lastly, *SDHA* mutations are a rare cause of PPGL and are classified as PGL5. They account for about 3% of cases and are also associated with GISTs and pituitary adenomas.[22,23]

Immunohistochemistry and Genetic Testing

The Endocrine Society Clinical Guidelines on Pheochromocytoma and Paraganglioma recommends that all patients with PPGL be engaged in shared decision-making for genetic testing as early knowledge of one's genetic status has a positive impact on management and clinical outcomes.[4,24] However, given the numerous PPGL susceptibility genes, traditional testing can be prohibitively costly and laborious. As such, the practice guidelines recommended tailoring testing for specific mutations based on the clinical presentation (ie, *RET* for those associated with medullary thyroid carcinoma, *VHL* for bilateral pheochromocytoma, *SDHx* for paragangliomas, *SDHB* for metastatic disease).[4] This limitation in conventional genetic testing was answered with the development of Next-Generation-Sequencing (NGS) which allowed for simultaneous testing of relevant genes in a single panel. This high throughput testing is most suitable for diseases with a diverse mutation pool like PPGL with studies suggesting that the use of NGS can reduce patient costs by lowering overall testing costs and reducing hospital visits.[25,26] Although genetic testing should be offered to all patients with PPGL, it is important to recognize financial, clinical, and psychological factors that may motivate their decision to pursue or delay testing. As such, it is the authors' practice and recommendation that patients offered genetic testing should first be seen by an expert genetic counselor to discuss the implication of testing for the patients and their family members.

When genetic testing is unavailable, immunohistochemical testing continues to have a place in the clinicians' diagnostic armamentarium.[27] SDHB and SDHA immunohistochemistry have shown to be reliable when identifying patients with *SDHx* mutations. Patients with *SDHB*, -*C*, and -*D* mutations develop tumors that are negative for SDHB immunostaining and positive for SDHA immunostaining, whereas patients with *SDHA* mutations have tumors negative for both SDHB and SDHA immunostaining. In a prospective study evaluating immunohistochemistry results for *SDHB*, *SDHC* and *SDHD* on 45 patients with PPGLs, the authors found that the sensitivity and specificity of the SDHB immunohistochemistry to detect the presence of an *SDHx* mutation were 100% and 84%, respectively.[28] However, routine use of immunohistochemical testing remains controversial because of interpretation variability and lower specificity, as in cases with SDHB weak diffuse staining, which can also be seen in those with VHL.[29]

PREOPERATIVE MANAGEMENT
Imaging

Preoperative imaging is invaluable for operative planning as it can localize a lesion, evaluate for multiplicity, and determine if there are synchronous metastases. Imaging modalities can be categorized into anatomic and functional imaging. Utilization of a combination of the two may help clinicians identify PPGLs.[4] Anatomic imaging primarily includes computed tomography (CT) and magnetic resonance imaging (MRI). Although there continues to be the development of novel, more sensitive radiotracers, common functional imaging includes metaiodobenzylguanidine (MIBG), ^{18}F-2-fluoro-2-deoxy-D-glucose (^{18}F-FDG PET), and more recently ^{68}Gallium-labeled (^{68}Ga) DOTATE PET/CT.[30]

Anatomic imaging provides excellent sensitivity in identifying potential PPGL lesions. Given the speed and excellent resolution, full body imaging with CT is usually sufficient and recommended over MRI.[4] However, MRI can be an appropriate alternative for those unable to have CT imaging (pregnant women, children, and those with contrast allergy). Although these modalities are extremely sensitive, limitations include false negative rates in the setting of metastatic disease and small PPGLs. As such, anatomic evaluation can be paired with functional imaging to improve the specificity as well as capture any missed lesions/metastasis.[4]

MIBG is historically the gold standard for functional imaging. However, the recent development of novel radiotracers has given other imaging modalities (^{18}F-FDG PET and ^{68}Ga-DOTATE PET/CT) superior sensitivity and resolution in identifying metastatic disease and paragangliomas.[31–34] If MIBG is considered, ^{123}I-MIBG should be used as it is more sensitive than ^{131}I-MIBG.[4] A unique benefit of using ^{123}I-MIBG is that it identifies tumors that are MIBG avid. This is of particular importance in those with metastatic/unresectable PPGL as high-specific-activity (HSA) ^{131}I-MIBG has shown promising results in controlling disease burden in these patients.[35] When looking specifically at patients with *SDHB* mutations, Timmers and colleagues[31,32] found that ^{18}F-FDG PET was superior to ^{123}I-MIBG and CT/MRI with a sensitivity approaching 100%, arguing that it should be the preferred imaging modality for staging *SDHB*-associated PPGLs. Most recently, there is a growing body of literature that demonstrates that (^{68}Ga)-DOTATE PET/CT is superior in detecting PPGL lesions compared with ^{18}F-FDG PET and CT/MRI (99% vs 86% vs 85%, respectively).[30] Optimal preoperative imaging remains unclear as more studies comparing contemporary radiotracers to conventional imaging modalities are needed.

Preoperative Blockade

Preoperative antihypertensive medication administration for PPGL surgery has been shown to decrease mortality/morbidity to rates less than 3% in retrospective studies.[36] The current recommendation from the Endocrine Society is for patients to undergo preoperative blockage with α-adrenergic receptor blockers first.[4] Studies have shown mixed results regarding whether selective or non-selective α-adrenergic receptor blockers are superior as initial antihypertensive therapy. In a recent randomized controlled clinical trial (RCT) including 134 patients with non-metastatic PPGL receiving phenoxybenzamine or doxazosin as preoperative hypertensive treatment, phenoxybenzamine was proven to be more effective than doxazosin in preventing intraoperative hemodynamic instability.[37] However, a previous retrospective study demonstrated that doxazosin is effective to lower preoperative diastolic blood pressure, intraoperative heart rate, and improve hemodynamic recovery, in addition to decreasing undesirable side effects like tachycardia.[38] The duration of preoperative antihypertensive treatment has also been debated. Kong and colleagues [39] analyzed perioperative hemodynamics and postoperative outcomes related to the duration of doxazosin therapy in 132 patients. Higher rates of intraoperative bradycardia and more postoperative hypotension requiring vasopressor support were documented when preoperative antihypertensive treatment was longer than 30 days. The recommendation by the Endocrine Society's guideline is to treat patients for 7 to 14 days to allow adequate time to normalize blood pressure and heart rate.[4]

The administration of α-adrenergic receptor blockers can have several clinically significant side effects including orthostatic, perioperative and postoperative hypotension sometimes requiring vasopressor support. Some recent studies have cited these potential side effects and the lack of a RCT demonstrating that antihypertensive premedication decreases morbidity/mortality as reasons to reevaluate the current premedication recommendations. Buisset and colleagues[40] described data on 134 patients undergoing unilateral adrenalectomy for pheochromocytoma for which 86% of the study cohort did not receive preoperative pharmacologic preparation. Cardiovascular morbidity was observed in 4.5% of patients with the main factor being the need for pressor amines postoperatively. Predictive factors of postoperative pressor amine use were tumor size, preoperative ß-blockers, and diuretics administration. In a multi-institutional study including 1860 patients with PPGLs, 343 of whom underwent surgical resection without α-blockade, the cardiovascular complication rate was significantly higher in patients with than in those without preoperative α-blockade (5.9%, 95% CI 4.7%–7.1% and 0.9%, 95% CI -0.1–1.9, respectively, $P < .001$). The mortality rate was similar among groups.[41] The availability of experienced anesthesiologists with good communication between the surgeon is likely the most important factor to manage the entire perioperative course effectively.

Some patients' hypertension and tachyarrhythmias are not completely controlled solely with α-adrenergic receptor blockers. In these patients, the administration of ß-adrenergic receptor blockers is indicated. However, it is extremely critical that ß-blockers not be administered before α-blockers have been properly adjusted because this would increase the risk of hypertension exacerbation.[42]

Alternative drugs for patients with poor tolerance to α-adrenergic receptor blockers are metyrosine and calcium channel blockers. Metyrosine, an inhibitor of the enzymatic activity of tyrosine hydroxylase, reduces catecholamine biosynthesis, reducing circulating catecholamine levels up to 80%. However, it is not widely available and can trigger adverse effects, particularly somnolence.[43] Calcium channel blockers are indicated as add-on drugs to improve blood pressure control in patients already being treated with α-adrenergic receptor blockers.[4]

SURGICAL MANAGEMENT
Indications and Objectives

Surgical resection remains the only potentially curative treatment for non-metastatic, SDHB-associated PPGLs. Any patient with known SDHB-associated PPGLs without absolute contraindications to surgery should be referred to an experienced surgeon for evaluation. The primary goals when treating hereditary PPGLs are (1) to provide symptom relief by removing the source of excess hormone secretion, (2) to prevent further growth, and (3) to minimize risk of recurrence and progression to metastatic disease.[44] Minimizing the risk of recurrence and development of metastatic disease cannot be underscored enough due to the high malignant potential specifically seen in SDHB-associated PPGLs. Currently, there are no biochemical, radiographic, or histologic characteristics that have been shown to accurately predict the likelihood of malignant behavior in these tumors. Patients are not infrequently referred to specialized centers years after initial resection for presumed sporadic disease, with some studies showing that metachronous lesions can be found as far as 20 years after index surgery.[12,45] As such, if features suggestive of potential malignant behavior (SDHB mutation, tumor size >5 cm, extra-adrenal location) are found preoperatively, patients should be evaluated and managed at a multidisciplinary care center with experts experienced in treating metastatic PPGLs to prevent the transformation of a potentially curable disease to an incurable one.[46,47] It is important to note that patients presenting with metastatic disease might not be excluded from surgery as removal of the primary tumor may slow disease progression (see Role of Surgery for Metastatic Pheochromocytomas and Paragangliomas section). Indeed, a study looking at overall survival using the Surveillance, Epidemiology, and End Results database, demonstrated that those who had no surgical intervention had worse overall survival.[48]

Surgical Approach

There are currently no prospective trials that have directly compared outcomes between laparoscopic and open approaches for SDHB-associated PPGL resection.

Although there are case reports of success with laparoscopic resection of small, noninvasive paragangliomas, given the higher risk of malignant behavior in *SDHB*-associated PPGL, experts recommend a cautious surgical approach to optimize complete resection without risking tumor rupture and seeding disease.[46,49] This is highlighted in a recent study by Nockel and colleagues[50] which looked at how preoperative genetic testing influenced surgical approach in PPGL resection. In that study, patients with an *SDHB* mutation were more likely to undergo open surgery compared with the rest of the cohort. This conservative approach is supported by later findings by Roman-Gonzalez *et al*[47] where patients with metastatic PPGL who underwent laparoscopic surgery had increased rates of local lymph node recurrence, which was also associated with shorter overall survival. Interestingly, Assadipour and colleagues[51] found that an open surgical approach was associated with increased local recurrence and distant metastasis. However, this finding is likely secondary to larger tumor sizes and extra-adrenal locations in patients undergoing open resection, both of which were also associated with increased local recurrence in their study.

Although laparoscopic surgery is lauded for bringing decreased postoperative pain and recovery times to patients, traditional open surgery offers unique advantages to experienced surgeons in these complex cases. Tactile evaluation of the tumor and surrounding structures can help intraoperative decision-making which can sometimes be dulled and/or non-existent in laparoscopic and robotic surgery. This is particularly important as studies suggest that occult lymph node metastasis may not be infrequent, as well as the fact that paragangliomas may be intimately associated with, or invading, major blood vessels (ie, aorta, inferior vena cava, and the superior mesenteric artery and vein).[52] In a retrospective case series of 29 patients with paragangliomas and major blood vessel involvement, Hu and colleagues[53] found that patients who underwent en bloc resection with vessel reconstruction had longer overall survival than those who simply underwent medical management. If there is concern for major blood vessel involvement, open surgery should be offered.

The decision on whether patients with familial PPGL should undergo a total versus cortical-sparing adrenalectomy, should depend on the mutation associated with the PPGL and the surgeons expertise. Cortical-sparing adrenalectomy was developed to preserve the ipsilateral, uninvolved adrenal cortex and has been shown to prevent adrenal insufficiency/crisis, has similarly low recurrence rates as total adrenalectomies, and is not associated with decreased survival.[54–56] This technique is largely used for patients with synchronous, or who have a genetic predisposition for developing bilateral pheochromocytomas (ie. MEN2, NF1 and VHL). However, this is a moot point as there have been no reports suggesting that patients with *SDHB* mutations have an increased risk of developing synchronous or metachronous bilateral pheochromocytomas. In fact, in a recent multicenter study including 625 patients with bilateral pheochromocytomas undergoing cortical-sparing adrenalectomy, only 1 of 526 patients with genetic testing had an *SDHB* mutation.[57] Adding to the complexity of treating *SDHB*-associated PPGL is that many cases of metastatic disease present as far back as 20 years after the index surgery for presumed benign disease.[45] Lastly, while experienced surgeons can differentiate cortex from adrenal medulla, there remains no intraoperative means to confidently confirm that all medullary cells are removed. As such, if a patient is found to have an *SDHB* mutation preoperatively, even in the setting of presumed benign, unilateral disease, all measures must be taken to decrease the risk of local regional recurrence and metastasis rather than preserving adrenal function. This is doubly true if the disease is found to have additional characteristics associated with malignancy (ie, tumor size >5 cm, extra-adrenal location).[4,44]

Lymph Node Dissection

Complete surgical resection (R0) should always be the primary objective for PPGL resection whenever feasible and safe. Although there is currently no study that has shown a survival benefit in patients who have had regional lymph node dissections, formal evaluation of surrounding lymph nodes may help accurately stage the patient. In a study by Abadin and colleagues[52] looking at subdiaphragmatic paragangliomas, incidental findings of lymph node metastatic deposits were not uncommon on final pathology. These findings can have prognostic significance as seen in the recently published 8th Edition AJCC staging system, where the presence of regional lymph node metastasis in patients with PPGL are upstaged to Stage III.[58] As mentioned previously, Roman-Gonzalez et al[47] found that two-thirds of patients with confirmed metastatic PPGLs had lymph node metastasis prompting them to suggest that patients who undergo surgery for PPGL with known clinical predictors of malignancy (ie, SDHB mutation), may benefit from concomitant lymph node dissection.

Role of Surgery for Metastatic Pheochromocytomas and Paragangliomas

Surgery also has a role in the management of metastatic PPGL. A study at MD Anderson by Roman-Gonzalez et al[47] found that resection of the primary tumor in patients with metastatic PPGL increased overall survival (148 months vs 36 months). Equally as important, palliative resection can provide symptomatic relief and improve the quality of life of patients suffering from hyperfunctioning tumors and those causing mass effect on adjacent organs. A caveat, however, is that while resection may objectively decrease the amount of antihypertensive medication needed, seldomly does it result in pharmacologic independence.[45,59] Furthermore, Ellis and colleagues[60,61] found that aggressive debulking purely for biochemical management was ineffective as few had partial biochemical improvement with the majority relapsing within 1 year.

Follow-up and Surveillance

All PPGL, regardless of genetic mutation status, have metastatic potential, and as such, mandate long-term follow-up. Professional societies suggest an individualized approach with at least 10 years of surveillance in all patients diagnosed with PPGLs.[62,63] In patients with high-risk characteristics for metastasis, lifelong biochemical testing is recommended with consideration for routine imaging to achieve the earliest detection of metastatic spread. Likewise, in those with an identified hereditary predisposition to PPGL, lifelong biochemical testing and imaging are indicated to identify metachronous tumor development. Although there is no consensus regarding using CT versus MRI for surveillance, if routine imaging will be incorporated into the patient's management plan, consider using or alternating CT with MRI to decrease radiation exposure.

SUMMARY

The growing list of mutations associated with pheochromocytoma and paraganglioma has made it increasingly clear that the maxim "rule of 10" underestimates the role of genetic analysis for these patients. Testing for and identification of patients with SDHB mutations will influence preoperative evaluation, operative planning, and postoperative surveillance. Patients with SDHB mutations require comprehensive biochemical testing and imaging to exclude synchronous metastatic disease. If feasible, these patients should undergo open surgery with the intent of complete surgical resection while minimizing the risk of locoregional recurrence and capsular rupture. Lastly, these patients need lifelong surveillance due to this disease's potentially long latency period for metachronous development. Patients who are preoperatively found to have an SDHB mutation or with high-risk features of metastatic potential should be evaluated and managed by a multidisciplinary team at specialized centers who are familiar with the intricacies of this complex disease.

CLINICS CARE POINTS

- All patients with pheochromocytomas and paragangliomas (PPGL) should undergo germline genetic testing as up to 40% of PPGL cases have an underlying mutation.
- Patients with succinate dehydrogenase subunit B (*SDHB*) mutations have a higher risk of developing synchronous and metachronous metastatic PPGL.
- Preoperative imaging is crucial to correctly stage PPGL patients and identify any synchronous metastasis. Functional imaging with novel radiotracers may become the optimal imaging modality for identifying *SDHB*-associated PPGLs and metastasis.
- As there is up to a 50% risk of malignancy, patients with *SDHB*-associated PPGL with worrisome imaging findings should undergo open, surgical resection when complete resection is feasible with the intention to minimize local regional recurrence and capsular rupture. Consider concurrent lymphadenectomy if there are any concerning regional lymph nodes.
- Patients with *SDHB* mutations will need lifelong surveillance with biochemical testing and consideration for routine imaging looking for recurrence and metachronous metastatic disease.

DISCLOSURE

This work is not supported by a specific funding source. The authors have no financial disclosures.

REFERENCES

1. Pacak K, Tella SH. Pheochromocytoma and Paraganglioma. In: Feingold KR, Anawalt B, Boyce A, et al., eds. Endotext. South Dartmouth (MA): MDText.com, Inc.Copyright © 2000-2022; 2000.
2. Jimenez C, Libutti S, Landry C, et al. AJCC cancer staging manual. New York, NY: Springer; 2016.
3. Buffet A, Burnichon N, Favier J, et al. An overview of 20 years of genetic studies in pheochromocytoma and paraganglioma. Best Pract Res Clin Endocrinol Metab 2020;34(2):101416.
4. Lenders JW, Duh QY, Eisenhofer G, et al. Pheochromocytoma and paraganglioma: an endocrine society clinical practice guideline. J Clin Endocrinol Metab 2014;99(6):1915–42.
5. Fishbein L, Leshchiner I, Walter V, et al. Comprehensive Molecular Characterization of Pheochromocytoma and Paraganglioma. Cancer Cell 2017;31(2):181–93.
6. Selak MA, Armour SM, MacKenzie ED, et al. Succinate links TCA cycle dysfunction to oncogenesis by inhibiting HIF-alpha prolyl hydroxylase. Cancer Cell 2005; 7(1):77–85.
7. Castro-Vega LJ, Buffet A, De Cubas AA, et al. Germline mutations in FH confer predisposition to malignant pheochromocytomas and paragangliomas. Hum Mol Genet 2014;23(9):2440–6.
8. Cascón A, Comino-Méndez I, Currás-Freixes M, et al. Whole-Exome Sequencing Identifies MDH2 as a New Familial Paraganglioma Gene. JNCI: J Natl Cancer Inst 2015;107(5).

9. Zhuang Z, Yang C, Lorenzo F, et al. Somatic HIF2A gain-of-function mutations in paraganglioma with polycythemia. N Engl J Med 2012;367(10):922–30.

10. Qin Y, Yao L, King EE, et al. Germline mutations in TMEM127 confer susceptibility to pheochromocytoma. Nat Genet 2010;42(3):229–33.

11. Comino-Méndez I, Gracia-Aznárez FJ, Schiavi F, et al. Exome sequencing identifies MAX mutations as a cause of hereditary pheochromocytoma. Nat Genet 2011;43(7):663–7.

12. Amar L, Bertherat J, Baudin E, et al. Genetic testing in pheochromocytoma or functional paraganglioma. J Clin Oncol 2005;23(34):8812–8.

13. Amar L, Baudin E, Burnichon N, et al. Succinate dehydrogenase B gene mutations predict survival in patients with malignant pheochromocytomas or paragangliomas. J Clin Endocrinol Metab 2007;92(10):3822–8.

14. Gimenez-Roqueplo AP, Favier J, Rustin P, et al. Mutations in the SDHB gene are associated with extra-adrenal and/or malignant phaeochromocytomas. Cancer Res 2003;63(17):5615–21.

15. Benn DE, Robinson BG, Clifton-Bligh RJ. 15 YEARS OF PARAGANGLIOMA: Clinical manifestations of paraganglioma syndromes types 1-5. Endocr Relat Cancer 2015;22(4):T91–103.

16. Benn DE, Gimenez-Roqueplo AP, Reilly JR, et al. Clinical presentation and penetrance of pheochromocytoma/paraganglioma syndromes. J Clin Endocrinol Metab 2006;91(3):827–36.

17. Neumann HP, Pawlu C, Peczkowska M, et al. Distinct clinical features of paraganglioma syndromes associated with SDHB and SDHD gene mutations. Jama 2004;292(8):943–51.

18. Schiavi F, Boedeker CC, Bausch B, et al. Predictors and prevalence of paraganglioma syndrome associated with mutations of the SDHC gene. Jama 2005;294(16):2057–63.

19. Kunst HP, Rutten MH, de Mönnink JP, et al. SDHAF2 (PGL2-SDH5) and hereditary head and neck paraganglioma. Clin Cancer Res 2011;17(2):247–54.

20. Brouwers FM, Eisenhofer G, Tao JJ, et al. High frequency of SDHB germline mutations in patients with malignant catecholamine-producing paragangliomas: implications for genetic testing. J Clin Endocrinol Metab 2006;91(11):4505–9.

21. Ricketts CJ, Forman JR, Rattenberry E, et al. Tumor risks and genotype-phenotype-proteotype analysis in 358 patients with germline mutations in SDHB and SDHD. Hum Mutat 2010;31(1):41–51.

22. Kopetschke R, Slisko M, Kilisli A, et al. Frequent incidental discovery of phaeochromocytoma: data from a German cohort of 201 phaeochromocytoma. Eur J Endocrinol 2009;161(2):355–61.

23. Dwight T, Benn DE, Clarkson A, et al. Loss of SDHA expression identifies SDHA mutations in succinate dehydrogenase-deficient gastrointestinal stromal tumors. Am J Surg Pathol 2013;37(2):226–33.

24. Buffet A, Ben Aim L, Leboulleux S, et al. Positive Impact of Genetic Test on the Management and Outcome of Patients With Paraganglioma and/or Pheochromocytoma. The J Clin Endocrinol Metab 2019;104(4):1109–18.

25. Toledo RA, Burnichon N, Cascon A, et al. Consensus Statement on next-generation-sequencing-based diagnostic testing of hereditary phaeochromocytomas and paragangliomas. Nat Rev Endocrinol 2017;13(4):233–47.

26. Pipitprapat W, Pattanaprateep O, Iemwimangsa N, et al. Cost-minimization analysis of sequential genetic testing versus targeted next-generation sequencing gene panels in patients with pheochromocytoma and paraganglioma. Ann Med 2021;53(1):1243–55.

27. Papathomas TG, Oudijk L, Persu A, et al. SDHB/SDHA immunohistochemistry in pheochromocytomas and paragangliomas: a multicenter interobserver variation analysis using virtual microscopy: a Multinational Study of the European Network for the Study of Adrenal Tumors (ENS@T). Mod Pathol 2015;28(6):807–21.
28. van Nederveen FH, Gaal J, Favier J, et al. An immunohistochemical procedure to detect patients with paraganglioma and phaeochromocytoma with germline SDHB, SDHC, or SDHD gene mutations: a retrospective and prospective analysis. Lancet Oncol 2009;10(8):764–71.
29. Gill AJ, Benn DE, Chou A, et al. Immunohistochemistry for SDHB triages genetic testing of SDHB, SDHC, and SDHD in paraganglioma-pheochromocytoma syndromes. Hum Pathol 2010;41(6):805–14.
30. Janssen I, Blanchet EM, Adams K, et al. Superiority of [68Ga]-DOTATATE PET/CT to Other Functional Imaging Modalities in the Localization of SDHB-Associated Metastatic Pheochromocytoma and Paraganglioma. Clin Cancer Res : official J Am Assoc Cancer Res 2015;21(17):3888–95.
31. Timmers HJ, Chen CC, Carrasquillo JA, et al. Staging and functional characterization of pheochromocytoma and paraganglioma by 18F-fluorodeoxyglucose (18F-FDG) positron emission tomography. J Natl Cancer Inst 2012;104(9):700–8.
32. Timmers HJ, Kozupa A, Chen CC, et al. Superiority of fluorodeoxyglucose positron emission tomography to other functional imaging techniques in the evaluation of metastatic SDHB-associated pheochromocytoma and paraganglioma. J Clin Oncol 2007;25(16):2262–9.
33. Bhatia KS, Ismail MM, Sahdev A, et al. 123I-metaiodobenzylguanidine (MIBG) scintigraphy for the detection of adrenal and extra-adrenal phaeochromocytomas: CT and MRI correlation. Clin Endocrinol (Oxf) 2008;69(2):181–8.
34. Wiseman GA, Pacak K, O'Dorisio MS, et al. Usefulness of 123I-MIBG scintigraphy in the evaluation of patients with known or suspected primary or metastatic pheochromocytoma or paraganglioma: results from a prospective multicenter trial. J Nucl Med 2009;50(9):1448–54.
35. Pryma DA, Chin BB, Noto RB, et al. Efficacy and Safety of High-Specific-Activity (131)I-MIBG Therapy in Patients with Advanced Pheochromocytoma or Paraganglioma. J Nucl Med 2019;60(5):623–30.
36. Livingstone M, Duttchen K, Thompson J, et al. Hemodynamic Stability During Pheochromocytoma Resection: Lessons Learned Over the Last Two Decades. Ann Surg Oncol 2015;22(13):4175–80.
37. Buitenwerf E, Osinga TE, Timmers H, et al. Efficacy of alpha-Blockers on Hemodynamic Control during Pheochromocytoma Resection: A Randomized Controlled Trial. J Clin Endocrinol Metab 2020;105(7).
38. Prys-Roberts C, Farndon JR. Efficacy and safety of doxazosin for perioperative management of patients with pheochromocytoma. World J Surg 2002;26(8):1037–42.
39. Kong H, Li N, Tian J, et al. The use of doxazosin before adrenalectomy for pheochromocytoma: is the duration related to intraoperative hemodynamics and postoperative complications? Int Urol Nephrol 2020;52(11):2079–85.
40. Buisset C, Guerin C, Cungi PJ, et al. Pheochromocytoma surgery without systematic preoperative pharmacological preparation: insights from a referral tertiary center experience. Surg Endosc 2021;35(2):728–35.
41. Groeben H, Walz MK, Nottebaum BJ, et al. International multicentre review of perioperative management and outcome for catecholamine-producing tumours. Br J Surg 2020;107(2):e170–8.

42. Sloand EM, Thompson BT. Propranolol-induced pulmonary edema and shock in a patient with pheochromocytoma. Arch Intern Med 1984;144(1):173–4.
43. Brogden RN, Heel RC, Speight TM, et al. alpha-Methyl-p-tyrosine: a review of its pharmacology and clinical use. Drugs 1981;21(2):81–9.
44. Jimenez C, Rohren E, Habra MA, et al. Current and future treatments for malignant pheochromocytoma and sympathetic paraganglioma. Curr Oncol Rep 2013;15(4):356–71.
45. Strajina V, Dy BM, Farley DR, et al. Surgical Treatment of Malignant Pheochromocytoma and Paraganglioma: Retrospective Case Series. Ann Surg Oncol 2017; 24(6):1546–50.
46. Ayala-Ramirez M, Feng L, Johnson MM, et al. Clinical risk factors for malignancy and overall survival in patients with pheochromocytomas and sympathetic paragangliomas: primary tumor size and primary tumor location as prognostic indicators. J Clin Endocrinol Metab 2011;96(3):717–25.
47. Roman-Gonzalez A, Zhou S, Ayala-Ramirez M, et al. Impact of Surgical Resection of the Primary Tumor on Overall Survival in Patients With Metastatic Pheochromocytoma or Sympathetic Paraganglioma. Ann Surg 2018;268(1):172–8.
48. Goffredo P, Sosa JA, Roman SA. Malignant pheochromocytoma and paraganglioma: a population level analysis of long-term survival over two decades. J Surg Oncol 2013;107(6):659–64.
49. Goers TA, Abdo M, Moley JF, et al. Outcomes of resection of extra-adrenal pheochromocytomas/paragangliomas in the laparoscopic era: a comparison with adrenal pheochromocytoma. Surg Endosc 2013;27(2):428–33.
50. Nockel P, El Lakis M, Gaitanidis A, et al. Preoperative genetic testing in pheochromocytomas and paragangliomas influences the surgical approach and the extent of adrenal surgery. Surgery 2018;163(1):191–6.
51. Assadipour Y, Sadowski SM, Alimchandani M, et al. SDHB mutation status and tumor size but not tumor grade are important predictors of clinical outcome in pheochromocytoma and abdominal paraganglioma. Surgery 2017;161(1):230–9.
52. Abadin SS, Ayala-Ramirez M, Jimenez C, et al. Impact of surgical resection for subdiaphragmatic paragangliomas. World J Surg 2014;38(3):733–41.
53. Hu H, Huang B, Zhao J, et al. En Bloc Resection with Major Blood Vessel Reconstruction for Locally Invasive Retroperitoneal Paragangliomas: A 15-Year Experience with Literature Review. World J Surg 2017;41(4):997–1004.
54. Yip L, Lee JE, Shapiro SE, et al. Surgical management of hereditary pheochromocytoma. J Am Coll Surg 2004;198(4):525–34 [discussion: 534-525].
55. Grubbs EG, Rich TA, Ng C, et al. Long-term outcomes of surgical treatment for hereditary pheochromocytoma. J Am Coll Surg 2013;216(2):280–9.
56. Castinetti F, Qi X-P, Walz MK, et al. Outcomes of adrenal-sparing surgery or total adrenalectomy in phaeochromocytoma associated with multiple endocrine neoplasia type 2: an international retrospective population-based study. The Lancet Oncol 2014;15(6):648–55.
57. Neumann HPH, Tsoy U, Bancos I, et al. Comparison of Pheochromocytoma-Specific Morbidity and Mortality Among Adults With Bilateral Pheochromocytomas Undergoing Total Adrenalectomy vs Cortical-Sparing Adrenalectomy. JAMA Netw Open 2019;2(8):e198898.
58. Amin M, Edge S, Greene F, et al. AJCC cancer staging manual. 8th edition. Springer International Publishing: American Joint Commission on Cancer; 2017.
59. Hamidi O, Young WF Jr, Iniguez-Ariza NM, et al. Malignant Pheochromocytoma and Paraganglioma: 272 Patients Over 55 Years. J Clin Endocrinol Metab 2017;102(9):3296–305.

60. Ellis RJ, Patel D, Prodanov T, et al. Response after surgical resection of metastatic pheochromocytoma and paraganglioma: can postoperative biochemical remission be predicted? J Am Coll Surg 2013;217(3):489–96.
61. Castinetti F, Taieb D, Henry JF, et al. MANAGEMENT OF ENDOCRINE DISEASE: Outcome of adrenal sparing surgery in heritable pheochromocytoma. Eur J Endocrinol 2016;174(1):R9–18.
62. Lenders JW, Duh QY, Eisenhofer G, et al. Pheochromocytoma and paraganglioma: an endocrine society clinical practice guideline. J Clin Endocrinol Metab 2014;99(6):1915–42.
63. Plouin PF, Amar L, Dekkers OM, et al. European Society of Endocrinology Clinical Practice Guideline for long-term follow-up of patients operated on for a phaeochromocytoma or a paraganglioma. Eur J Endocrinol 2016;174(5):G1–10.

Genetic Testing for Adrenal Tumors—What the Contemporary Surgeon Should Know

Maria F. Bates, MD[a,b,c], Meredith J. Sorensen, MD, MS[a,b,c],*

KEYWORDS

• Adrenal • Genetic testing • Adrenalectomy • Familial syndromes

KEY POINTS

- Familial syndromes exist in many surgical adrenal diseases.
- Genetic testing is available and referral to genetic counselor should be considered for most adrenal diseases.
- Germline mutation testing can help guide perioperative management, postoperative risk assessment, postoperative follow-up, and screening of family members.

INTRODUCTION

In the last few decades, there have been many scientific advances in genetics, including the sequencing of the entire human genome in 2003.[1] Shortly afterward, next-generation sequencing (NGS), a high-throughput DNA sequencing, became commercially available, allowing for rapid and cost-efficient methods used to sequence targeted gene panels.[2] These advances have led to the identification of more germline mutations in various diseases. In the field of adrenal medicine, the surgical diseases include pheochromocytoma (PCC), paragangliomas (PGLs), primary hyperaldosteronism, Cushing syndrome, and adrenocortical carcinoma (ACC). Familial syndromes are associated with all of these conditions, and multiple germline mutations have been identified. As medicine advances, more and more mutations are discovered each year. Historically, for example, only 10% of PCCs were thought to be familial; now it is thought that up to 40% of patients with this disease have a

[a] Geisel School of Medicine at Dartmouth, Hanover, NH, USA; [b] Department of Surgery, Dartmouth-Hitchcock Medical Center, Lebanon, NH 03756, USA; [c] Section of General Surgery, Division of Endocrine Surgery, One Medical Center Drive, Lebanon, NH 03756, USA
* Corresponding author.
E-mail address: Meredith.J.Sorensen@hitchcock.org
Twitter: @mfbates13 (M.F.B.); @MJSorensenMD (M.J.S.)

Surg Oncol Clin N Am 32 (2023) 303–313
https://doi.org/10.1016/j.soc.2022.10.007

germline mutation.[3,4] With these evolving discoveries, it is even more important for the adrenal surgeon to be familiar with the associated familial syndromes in surgical adrenal diseases. Identification of patients with familial syndromes allows for the detection and screening of associated syndromic neoplasms, guides surgical planning and operative approach, influences recurrence and malignancy risk assessment, aids in the development of postoperative surveillance plans, and determines the need for screening family members. Here, we review the major familial syndromes associated with adrenal surgical diseases and discuss currently available genetic testing and treatment recommendations.

PHEOCHROMOCYTOMA AND PARAGANGLIOMA
Background

PCC and PGLs are both catecholamine-secreting tumors. PCCs are located within the adrenal medulla of the adrenal gland, whereas PGLs are in extra-adrenal locations, found anywhere along the sympathetic chain from the neck to the pelvis. These 2 tumors have similar behaviors clinically and therefore clinical treatments are similar. However, it is important to distinguish between the 2 because there are slight differences in the risk of associated neoplasms, the risk for malignancy or metastatic spread, and the genetic basis.

Originally, PCCs and PGLs were considered to be 10% familial but now up to 40% of cases are associated with known mutations.[3,4] In general, patients with familial disease present at an earlier age and have a higher chance of bilateral disease or multifocal disease. More than 20 genes have been found to play a role in tumor development, either as germline or as somatic mutations.[5] Consequently, recommendations have recently changed in the last decade and current consensus is to refer all patients with these tumor types for genetic testing.[4] It is important to determine if the condition is part of a familial syndrome because the genetic basis of the disease may guide surgical decision-making, risk of other syndrome-associated tumors, risk of recurrence, help establish a surveillance plan, and decide whether family members should be screened.

Familial Syndromes Associated with Pheochromocytoma and Paraganglioma

Multiple endocrine neoplasia type 2
Patients with multiple endocrine neoplasia type 2 (MEN2) carry an autosomal dominant mutation in the RET proto-oncogene. There are 2 primary subtypes, MEN2A and MEN2B, with MEN2A making up 95% of MEN2 syndromes. In MEN2A, 100% of patients present with medullary thyroid carcinoma (MTC), 50% develop PCC (which are bilateral 50% of the time but rarely malignant), and ~20% also develop parathyroid hyperplasia. In MEN2B, patients also present with MTC and PCC but with mucocutaneous neuromas rather than parathyroid disease. Most of the MEN2 patients diagnosed with catecholamine-secreting tumors have a PCC rather than a PGL.

Von hippel-lindau
Von hippel-lindau (VHL) is inherited via an autosomal dominant mutation in the VHL tumor suppressor gene. This syndrome is associated with CNS hemangioblastomas, pancreatic neuroendocrine tumors, and renal cell carcinomas in addition to PCCs/PGLs. There are various types of VHL but only type II variants are associated with PCCs/PGLs. 20% of patients with VHL develop a PCC or PGL. They are generally noradrenergic tumors and can be in the abdomen, mediastinum, or pelvis. These tumors are rarely malignant, often develop in the younger population (with a mean age of

diagnosis of 30 years) and may be adrenal or extra-adrenal. Recurrence in patients with VHL is more common than those with sporadic PCCs.[6]

Neurofibromatosis type 1
Again, this syndrome has autosomal dominant inheritance and involves a mutation in the tumor suppressor gene neurofibromatosis type 1 (NF1). It classically presents with café-au-lait spots, mucocutaneous neurofibromas, inguinal or axillary freckling, Lisch nodules, optic nerve gliomas, and long bone dysplasia. In addition, 3% of people with NF1 will develop a unilateral PCC, up to 12% of which are malignant.[7] Any patient with NF1 and hypertension should undergo screening for PCC.

SDHx syndromes
SDHx syndromes, also known as the paraganglioma syndromes, are caused by mutations in the succinate dehydrogenase (SDH) complex. Most familial PGLs are caused by SDH complex mutations. There are 5 associated types: SDHA, SDHB, SDHC, SDHD, and SDHAF2. Most of these mutations will cause PGLs; however, PCCs are seen in all 5 subtypes as well. Most importantly, SDHB mutation has a 30% to 70% risk of these patients developing malignant PGL/PCC.[8]

Carney triad
Carney Triad is a familial syndrome made of gastrointestinal stromal tumors, PGLs, and pulmonary chondromas. Less commonly, these patients can also develop adrenocortical adenomas, PCCs, and esophageal leiomyomas. The Carney triad mostly affects younger women, and the onset is usually the second decade of life or later. It is thought that the syndrome is caused by downregulation of the SDH enzyme complex though site-specific hypermethylation of the SDHC gene.[9]

Genetic Testing

Traditionally, it was recommended that patients should undergo genetic testing if they had any of the following: diagnosis of PGL, bilateral PCC, unilateral PCC with family history of PCC/PGL, unilateral PCC with age less than 45 years, or other clinical findings of associated syndromic disorders. Recently recommendations have changed, and the new consensus is that everyone with a PCC or PGL should be tested for germline mutations.[10,11] Up to 40% of PCCs/PGLs have germline mutations, and up to 20% of those occur in patients without a family history, previously thought to be sporadic.[12] NGS is now the gold standard for genetic testing and sequence analysis because it is efficient and cost-effective. NGS makes it easy to test for 10 to 20 of the most common genes associated with familial PCCs/PGLs.[5]

Treatment

The standard of care for PCCs and PGLs is surgical resection when feasible. The presence of a germline mutation or associated syndrome can affect surgical decision-making and surgical approach to PCCs and PGLs. For example, patients identified with an SDHB mutation often will undergo open resection due to the malignancy potential.[13] Cortical-sparing adrenalectomy is considered in patients with MEN2 or VHL because of the risk for bilateral disease.[14] This approach helps avoid adrenal insufficiency in most patients but also increases the risk of recurrence. Because of this, patients and providers should weigh the risks and benefits of each surgical approach and assess the patient preferences.

Clinics Care Points

- At least 40% of PCCs and PGLs are familial.

- Familial syndromes with PCC and PGL include MEN2, VHL, NF1, SDHx syndromes, and Carney Triad.
- All patients with PCC and PGL should undergo genetic testing.
- Diagnosis of associated familial syndromes can affect surgical approach as well as surveillance recommendations.

PRIMARY HYPERALDOSTERONISM
Background

Primary hyperaldosteronism, also known as Conn syndrome,[15] is a disorder that leads to excessive and autonomous aldosterone production. This leads to a clinical syndrome of high blood pressure, often presenting at an early age, and usually requires multiple antihypertensive agents to treat. Approximately half the patients also present with hypokalemia. The most common causes for primary hyperaldosteronism are single adrenal adenoma, unilateral adrenal hyperplasia, or bilateral adrenal hyperplasia. In less common situations, primary hyperaldosteronism is caused by an ACC or inherited conditions of familial hyperaldosteronism.[16] Although the first-line treatment of familial hyperaldosteronism is typically not adrenalectomy, it is important for surgeons to be aware of these familial syndromes to appropriately diagnose and treat this select group of patients.

Familial Primary Hyperaldosteronism

There are 4 types of familial primary hyperaldosteronism (**Table 1**). All follow a pattern of autosomal dominant inheritance. Familial hyperaldosteronism type I, also known as glucocorticoid remediable aldosteronism (GRA),[16] makes up 1% of cases of primary hyperaldosteronism.[17] It is caused by a mutation in 2 genes, which results in chimeric gene fusion CYP11B1/CYP11B2 complex leads to endogenous adrenocorticotropic hormone (ACTH) secretion and hypersecretion of aldosterone. The phenotypic presentation can vary from mild disease to severe hypertension refractory to medical management.[17] Familial hyperaldosteronism type II accounts for less than 6% of patients with primary hyperaldosteronism. The exact molecular basis is unclear, and it is thought to involve multiple genetic steps.[16] Recent studies demonstrate association with chromosomal region 7p22,[18] as well as a CLCN2 chloride channel mutation.[19] Familial hyperaldosteronism type III often presents clinically before the age of 20 and also can be mild to severe. It is caused by a mutation in the KCNJ5 gene, which encodes the potassium channel Kir 3.4.[20] This mutation indirectly leads to calcium influx resulting in aldosterone production and cell proliferation. Type IV familial hyperaldosteronism is also known as early onset primary hyperaldosteronism and presents with seizures and neurologic abnormalities. It is due to a mutation in the CACNA1H

Table 1 Familial primary hyperaldosteronism		
Type Familial Primary Hyperaldosteronism	**Genetic Mutations**	**Treatment**
FH – I	CYP11B1/CYP11B2	Glucocorticoids
FH – II	CLCN2	MRA
FH – III	KCNJ5	MRA ± Adrenalectomy
FH – IV	CACNA1H	MRA ± Adrenalectomy

Abbreviation: MRA, mineralocorticoid receptor antagonist.

gene, which encodes a subunit of a voltage-gated calcium channel.[21] Although its inheritance is autosomal dominant, it demonstrates incomplete penetrance.

Genetic Testing

Genetic testing for familial hyperaldosteronism should be considered in a subset of patients.
The following individuals should be tested:

- Diagnosis of primary hyperaldosteronism at less than 20 years of age
- Family history of primary hyperaldosteronism
- Family history of stroke at young age (less than 40 years of age)
- Children or young adults with severe or resistant hypertension and positive family history of early onset hypertension and/or premature hemorrhagic stroke

Genetic testing for familial hyperaldosteronism is done via a familial hyperaldosteronism panel that includes Southern blot or PCR for the CYP11B1/CYP11B2 mutation (very sensitive and specific for FH-I/GRA),[16] testing for CLCN2 mutations (type-II), germline mutations in KCNJ5 (type-III), and CACNA1H mutations (type-IV).[22]

Treatment

Most of the familial hyperaldosteronism syndromes are treated medically; however, surgical adrenalectomy is sometimes indicated. Patients with familial hyperaldosteronism type III and type IV can develop severe bilateral adrenal hyperplasia. Initial treatment is medical with mineralocorticoid receptor antagonists (MRA). Occasionally, disease refractory to MRAs can be severe enough that bilateral adrenalectomy is indicated.[23]

Clinics Care Points

- There are 4 types of familial hyperaldosteronism.
- All are autosomal dominant.
- Genetic testing should be considered in patients diagnosed age younger than 20 years, with family history of hyperaldosteronism or stroke at age younger than 40 years, or children with severe or resistant hypertension and positive family history of early onset hypertension or premature hemorrhagic stroke.
- Management of familial hyperaldosteronism is typically medical but the disease can be severe enough in type III/IV that bilateral adrenalectomy is indicated.

CORTISOL-PRODUCING ADRENAL SYNDROMES
Background

Cushing syndrome results in cortisol excess in the body. It is caused by either an excess of pituitary or ectopic ACTH or ACTH-independent cortisol production by an adrenocortical adenoma or carcinoma or adrenal hyperplasia. Adrenal adenomas are responsible for 10% to 15% of all cases of Cushing syndrome, with ACCs making up less than 5%. Somatic mutations in the PRKACA gene, which encodes a catalytic subunit of cAMP-dependent protein kinase A (PKA), is the underlying somatic mutation in approximately 50% of adrenal adenomas that cause overt Cushing syndrome.[24] However, a very small subset of Cushing syndrome is caused by ACTH-independent familial syndromes that result in bilateral adrenal hyperplasia.

Familial Syndromes

Carney complex

The Carney complex is a variant of primary pigmented nodular adrenal hyperplasia (PPNAD). It is a familial syndrome with autosomal dominant inheritance. PPNAD is characterized by ACTH-independent bilateral adrenal hyperplasia with pigmented adrenal micronodules. In addition to Cushing syndrome, Carney complex can present with mesenchymal tumors such as atrial myxoma, spotty skin pigmentation, peripheral nerve tumors, breast lesions, testicular tumors, and GH-secreting pituitary tumors.[25] Patients with Carney complex usually present with Cushing syndrome by age 30, and 50% of patients are aged younger than 15 years when diagnosed.[26] The underlying genetic cause of Carney complex is variable, with more than 135 mutations identified, most of which are germline mutations. The cAMP-PKA signaling pathway is the main area involved in the molecular pathogenesis of this syndrome.[27] Mutations in the PKA regulatory subunit type IA (PRKAR1A) gene lead to abnormal PKA signaling.[28] This mutation has been identified in 70% of patients with Carney complex.[27] The biochemical diagnosis of Carney complex confirms ACTH-independent cortisol excess from the adrenal glands. Caution must be taken when relying on cross-sectional imaging to support the diagnosis because the adrenal glands often seem normal or only slightly enlarged.

Primary macronodular adrenal hyperplasia

These patients present with ACTH-independent bilateral adrenal hyperplasia with macronodules. Functionally, they can have various levels of cortisol secretion, leading to variable clinical presentations. In primary macronodular adrenal hyperplasia (PMAH), cortisol synthesis is not stimulated by ACTH. Instead, it is regulated by aberrant hormonal receptors in the adrenal cortex, such as MC2R gene, PRKACA, and PDE11 A.[29] When these are coupled to G-proteins, they activate the cAMP-PKA pathway, leading to steroid production and adrenal hyperplasia. In contrast to PPNAD, the adrenal nodules are large and can lead to massively enlarged adrenal glands. Multiple genetic mutations are hypothesized to cause this syndrome. Both germline and somatic mutations have been linked to PMAH. The most common mutation is in the ARMC5 gene, a tumor suppressor gene, believed to contribute to more than 80% of familial forms of PMAH and 30% of sporadic cases.[30,31] PMAH is also seen in other types of familial syndromes including MEN1, FAP, and HLRCC (hereditary leiomyomatosis and renal cell cancer).

Genetic Testing

For patients with Carney complex, genetic counseling and testing for PRKAR1A gene mutations should be considered. Patients with PMAH, especially those with severe Cushing syndrome and massively enlarged adrenal glands, should consider genetic counseling and testing for ARMC5 gene mutations.[32]

Treatment

In general, treatment includes both medical and surgical approaches. Treatment should be considered for patients with mild autonomous cortisol production with associated comorbidities (ie, osteoporosis, diabetes), as well as those with overt and severe Cushing syndrome.

Medical treatment includes the steroid synthesis inhibitors ketoconazole and metyrapone. These are used when surgery is not possible and for those with mild autonomous cortisol production and no associated comorbidities.

For both Carney complex and PMAH, bilateral adrenalectomy is curative. However, this results in adrenal insufficiency and requires lifelong steroid replacement. Therefore, unilateral or subtotal adrenalectomy may be considered. Steroid production often correlates with adrenal size, so one can consider debulking the glands.[32] Unilateral adrenalectomy may be reasonable if there is one dominant gland. Total unilateral adrenalectomy of the largest gland with partial adrenalectomy of the contralateral gland is another approach. Both are reasonable surgical options in patients with mild hypercortisolism and associated cortisol-excess comorbidities or in patients likely to be noncompliant with lifelong steroid replacement.[31]

Clinics Care Points

- Cushing syndrome is due to familial syndromes in a small percentage of patients.
- The 2 associated syndromes are Carney complex, a variant of PPNAD, and PMAH.
- Patients with adrenal Cushing syndrome and other syndromic features should be referred for genetic testing.
- Adrenalectomy (either bilateral total or subtotal) is the recommended treatment of those with associated secondary comorbidities related to cortisol excess and those with overt or severe Cushing syndrome.

ADRENOCORTICAL CARCINOMA
Background

ACC is a primary malignant tumor of the adrenal cortex. Although this disease is rare, it is often an aggressive tumor with an overall 5-year survival rate in all stages of 50%. Approximately 5% to 10% of ACCs are associated with germline mutations and are associated with many familial cancer syndromes in adults, including multiple endocrine neoplasia type I (MEN-1), familial adenomatous polyposis (FAP), and Lynch syndrome.[33,34] In contrast, 60% to 80% of children with ACC have an associated germline mutation, often Li Fraumeni syndrome (LFS) and Beckwith Wiedemann syndrome (BWS).[35]

Familial Syndromes Associated with Adrenocortical Carcinoma

MEN1: Approximately, 1% to 2% of patients with ACC have MEN1 mutation.[36] The patients usually also have primary hyperparathyroidism, pancreatic neuroendocrine tumors, and/or pituitary adenomas. Up to 73% of patients with MEN1 develop adrenal enlargement and/or adenomas, depending on radiological methods and criteria used to define adrenal enlargement.[37] In one study of 715 patients with MEN1, 13.8% of these patients were diagnosed with ACC.[36] Annual abdominal imaging should be done in this patient population for neuroendocrine tumor surveillance but should also be done because of the high rate of ACCs in this syndrome. Any adrenal lesion identified on surveillance imaging needs dedicated adrenal radiographic studies as well as formal adrenal hormonal evaluation.[33]

FAP (Gardner syndrome): This syndrome is due to mutations in the APC gene, a tumor suppressor gene. Approximately 7% to 13% of FAP patients develop adrenocortical adenomas, compared with less than 5% in the general population.[38] Although the colorectal and adrenal adenomas have similar malignant potential, patients with FAP develop hundreds to thousands of colorectal adenomas but only 1 or 2 adrenal adenomas.[33] As a result, the ACC risk in patients with FAP is very low compared with the risk of colorectal cancer. For this reason, regular screening for ACC in patients with FAP is not recommended.

Lynch Syndrome (hereditary nonpolyposis colorectal cancer HNPCC): This autosomal dominant syndrome is caused by mutations in the mismatch repair genes: *MLH1*, *MSH2*, *MSH6*, *PMS2*, and *EPCAM*. Patients with Lynch syndrome have a high risk of colon cancer (20%–80%). Other associated neoplasms include, uterine, gastric, ovarian, small bowel, pancreatic, prostate, kidney, bile duct, brain, urinary tract, and adrenal. The incidence of adrenal neoplasms in Lynch syndrome is 3.2%. In one series of 94 patients with ACC, 3 tested positive for Lynch syndrome with mismatch repair gene mutations.[39] The screening test for Lynch syndrome is done on tumor tissue by performing microsatellite instability testing and immunohistochemistry testing. For patients who have undergone resection for ACC, it is recommended to perform these 2 screening tests on the tumor, which will help determine if more specific genetic testing is necessary.[33] Lynch syndrome-associated colorectal carcinoma has an increased response to immunotherapy, suggesting that there may also be a role for immunotherapy in Lynch syndrome-associated ACCs.[33]

Li Fraumeni syndrome: About 70% of patients diagnosed with LFS have a mutation in the Tp53 gene.[35] ACCs usually are the presenting cancer and most often present in childhood. In general, any ACC diagnosed in a child should raise suspicion for a germline mutation and an associated cancer syndrome. Patients with LFS can also present with osteosarcoma, sarcoma, acute leukemia, breast cancer, brain cancer, melanoma, and colon cancer.[40]

Beckwith-Wiedemann syndrome: This syndrome causes increased cancer risk in childhood and is due mostly to alterations on chromosome 11 in the IGF2 gene. One percent of children with BWS will get an ACC in childhood. Interestingly, the risk of developing an ACC tapers off by adulthood.[33]

Table 2 lists the frequency of ACC in each of the associated syndromes.

Genetic Testing

All children who are diagnosed with ACC should undergo genetic screening, specifically for LFS. For adults with ACC, genetic testing should also be considered and should also include testing for LFS and LS.[33] For all other syndromes, the syndrome diagnosis is often already established at the time of ACC diagnosis. Established ACC programs recommend an algorithm including genetic counseling, a 4-generation pedigree, a review of personal medical history, a physical examination, and screening of ACC tumor tissue for the absence of DNA mismatch repair proteins (Lynch syndrome). FAP and NF1 are often diagnosed on clinical examination. Direct germline testing for MSH2, MSH6, PMS2, MLH1, EPCAM, MEN1, APC, and TP53 should be offered to all patients with ACC.[33] It is important to perform genetic testing in these patients because it can help establish a surveillance plan for each patient, lead to

Table 2		
Frequency and presentation of adrenocortical carcinoma and associated familial syndromes[33]		
Syndrome	Percentage of Patients with ACC	Time of Presentation
Li-Fraumeni syndrome	2%–4%	Childhood
Lynch syndrome	3%	Adulthood
MEN1 syndrome	1%–2%	Adulthood
Familial adenomatous polyposis	<1%	Adulthood
Beckwith-Wiedemann	<1%	Childhood

earlier diagnosis and earlier treatment of other syndrome-associated neoplasms, and help identify and screen family members at risk.

Treatment

Treatment of ACC with associated familial syndromes is the same as for sporadic ACC. If resectable, open adrenalectomy with en bloc resection of surrounding organs and/or lymphadenectomy is recommended. In patients with Lynch syndrome, radiation should be avoided due to increased risk of secondary malignancies.[41]

Clinics Care Points

- Familial syndromes are associated with ACC in 5% to 10% of adults and 60% to 80% of children.
- The most common syndromes are MEN1, FAP, LS, LFS, and BWS.
- All patients with ACC should undergo targeted genetic testing.
- Syndrome diagnosis helps surveil for other associated neoplasms, aids in developing a surveillance plan, and helps screen at-risk family.

SUMMARY

All surgical diseases of the adrenal gland are associated with familial syndromes to varying degrees. With the advancement of DNA sequencing and molecular analysis leading to the discovery of more germline mutations, these familial associations will likely continue to increase in prevalence. Knowledge of these syndromes is essential for the adrenal surgeon. Most patients with adrenal pathologic condition should be considered for targeted genetic testing, or at least referral for genetic counseling. Diagnosis of a familial syndrome is helpful in the perioperative period for determining surgical approach, extent of surgery, recurrence risk, and malignancy risk. It also aids in developing a long-term surveillance plan for each patient. Finally, it allows us to identify at-risk family members, potentially leading to earlier diagnosis, earlier treatment, and ultimately better outcomes.

DISCLOSURE

The authors have nothing to disclose.

REFERENCES

1. Hood L, Rowen L. The Human Genome Project: big science transforms biology and medicine. Genome Med 2013;5(9):79.
2. Rizzo JM, Buck MJ. Key principles and clinical applications of "next-generation" DNA sequencing. Cancer Prev Res Phila Pa 2012;5(7):887–900.
3. Fishbein L. Pheochromocytoma and Paraganglioma: Genetics, Diagnosis, and Treatment. Hematol Oncol Clin North Am 2016;30(1):135–50.
4. Alrezk R, Suarez A, Tena I, et al. Update of Pheochromocytoma Syndromes: Genetics, Biochemical Evaluation, and Imaging. Front Endocrinol 2018;9:515.
5. Patel D, Phay JE, Yen TWF, et al. Update on Pheochromocytoma and Paraganglioma from the SSO Endocrine/Head and Neck Disease-Site Work Group. Part 1 of 2: Advances in Pathogenesis and Diagnosis of Pheochromocytoma and Paraganglioma. Ann Surg Oncol 2020;27(5):1329–37.
6. Li SR, Nicholson KJ, Mccoy KL, et al. Clinical and Biochemical Features of Pheochromocytoma Characteristic of Von Hippel-Lindau Syndrome. World J Surg 2020;44(2):570–7.

7. Gruber LM, Erickson D, Babovic-Vuksanovic D, et al. Pheochromocytoma and paraganglioma in patients with neurofibromatosis type 1. Clin Endocrinol (Oxf) 2017;86(1):141–9.
8. Lefebvre M, Foulkes WD. Pheochromocytoma and paraganglioma syndromes: genetics and management update. Curr Oncol Tor Ont 2014;21(1):e8–17.
9. Settas N, Faucz FR, Stratakis CA. Succinate dehydrogenase (SDH) deficiency, Carney triad and the epigenome. Mol Cell Endocrinol 2018;469:107–11.
10. Plouin PF, Amar L, Dekkers OM, et al. European Society of Endocrinology Clinical Practice Guideline for long-term follow-up of patients operated on for a phaeochromocytoma or a paraganglioma. Eur J Endocrinol 2016;174(5):G1–10.
11. Lenders JWM, Duh QY, Eisenhofer G, et al. Pheochromocytoma and paraganglioma: an endocrine society clinical practice guideline. J Clin Endocrinol Metab 2014;99(6):1915–42.
12. Kim JH, Kim MJ, Kong SH, et al. Characteristics of germline mutations in Korean patients with pheochromocytoma/paraganglioma. J Med Genet 2022;59(1):56–64.
13. Nockel P, El Lakis M, Gaitanidis A, et al. Preoperative genetic testing in pheochromocytomas and paragangliomas influences the surgical approach and the extent of adrenal surgery. Surgery 2018;163(1):191–6.
14. Patel D, Phay JE, Yen TWF, et al. Update on Pheochromocytoma and Paraganglioma from the SSO Endocrine and Head and Neck Disease Site Working Group, Part 2 of 2: Perioperative Management and Outcomes of Pheochromocytoma and Paraganglioma. Ann Surg Oncol 2020;27(5):1338–47.
15. Conn JW. The evolution of primary aldosteronism: 1954-1967. Harvey Lect 1966;62:257–91.
16. Funder JW, Carey RM, Mantero F, et al. The Management of Primary Aldosteronism: Case Detection, Diagnosis, and Treatment: An Endocrine Society Clinical Practice Guideline. J Clin Endocrinol Metab 2016;101(5):1889–916.
17. Mulatero P, Tizzani D, Viola A, et al. Prevalence and characteristics of familial hyperaldosteronism: the PATOGEN study (Primary Aldosteronism in TOrino-GENetic forms). Hypertens Dallas Tex 1979 2011;58(5):797–803.
18. So A, Duffy DL, Gordon RD, et al. Familial hyperaldosteronism type II is linked to the chromosome 7p22 region but also shows predicted heterogeneity. J Hypertens 2005;23(8):1477–84.
19. Fernandes-Rosa FL, Daniil G, Orozco IJ, et al. A gain-of-function mutation in the CLCN2 chloride channel gene causes primary aldosteronism. Nat Genet 2018;50(3):355–61.
20. Choi M, Scholl UI, Yue P, et al. K+ channel mutations in adrenal aldosterone-producing adenomas and hereditary hypertension. Science 2011;331(6018):768–72.
21. Melmed S, Polonsky K, Larsen P, Kronenberg H. (2016) Williams Textbook of Endocrinology. 13th edition. Elsevier.
22. NIH - GTR: Genetic Testing Registry. Available at: https://www.ncbi.nlm.nih.gov/gtr/. Accessed July 7, 2022.
23. Geller DS, Zhang J, Wisgerhof MV, et al. A novel form of human mendelian hypertension featuring nonglucocorticoid-remediable aldosteronism. J Clin Endocrinol Metab 2008;93(8):3117–23.
24. Beuschlein F, Fassnacht M, Assié G, et al. Constitutive activation of PKA catalytic subunit in adrenal Cushing's syndrome. N Engl J Med 2014;370(11):1019–28.

25. Salpea P, Stratakis CA. Carney complex and McCune Albright syndrome: an overview of clinical manifestations and human molecular genetics. Mol Cell Endocrinol 2014;386(1–2):85–91.
26. Young WF, Carney JA, Musa BU, et al. Familial Cushing's syndrome due to primary pigmented nodular adrenocortical disease. Reinvestigation 50 years later. N Engl J Med 1989;321(24):1659–64.
27. Tirosh A, Valdés N, Stratakis CA. Genetics of micronodular adrenal hyperplasia and Carney complex. Presse Medicale Paris Fr 1983 2018;47(7–8 Pt 2):e127–37.
28. Kirschner LS, Carney JA, Pack SD, et al. Mutations of the gene encoding the protein kinase A type I-alpha regulatory subunit in patients with the Carney complex. Nat Genet 2000;26(1):89–92.
29. Christopoulos S, Bourdeau I, Lacroix A. Aberrant expression of hormone receptors in adrenal Cushing's syndrome. Pituitary 2004;7(4):225–35.
30. Assié G, Libé R, Espiard S, et al. ARMC5 mutations in macronodular adrenal hyperplasia with Cushing's syndrome. N Engl J Med 2013;369(22):2105–14.
31. Charchar HLS, Fragoso MCBV. An Overview of the Heterogeneous Causes of Cushing Syndrome Resulting From Primary Macronodular Adrenal Hyperplasia (PMAH). J Endocr Soc 2022;6(5):bvac041.
32. Bouys L, Chiodini I, Arlt W, et al. Update on primary bilateral macronodular adrenal hyperplasia (PBMAH). Endocrine 2021;71(3):595–603.
33. Petr EJ, Else T. Adrenocortical carcinoma (ACC): When and why should we consider germline testing? Presse Medicale Paris Fr 1983 2018;47(7–8 Pt 2): e119–25.
34. Else T. Association of adrenocortical carcinoma with familial cancer susceptibility syndromes. Mol Cell Endocrinol 2012;351(1):66–70.
35. Rodriguez-Galindo C, Figueiredo BC, Zambetti GP, et al. Biology, clinical characteristics, and management of adrenocortical tumors in children. Pediatr Blood Cancer 2005;45(3):265–73.
36. Gatta-Cherifi B, Chabre O, Murat A, et al. Adrenal involvement in MEN1. Analysis of 715 cases from the Groupe d'etude des Tumeurs Endocrines database. Eur J Endocrinol 2012;166(2):269–79.
37. Schaefer S, Shipotko M, Meyer S, et al. Natural course of small adrenal lesions in multiple endocrine neoplasia type 1: an endoscopic ultrasound imaging study. Eur J Endocrinol 2008;158(5):699–704.
38. Smith TG, Clark SK, Katz DE, et al. Adrenal masses are associated with familial adenomatous polyposis. Dis Colon Rectum 2000;43(12):1739–42.
39. Raymond VM, Everett JN, Furtado LV, et al. Adrenocortical carcinoma is a lynch syndrome-associated cancer. J Clin Oncol Off J Am Soc Clin Oncol 2013;31(24): 3012–8.
40. Ruijs MWG, Verhoef S, Rookus MA, et al. TP53 germline mutation testing in 180 families suspected of Li-Fraumeni syndrome: mutation detection rate and relative frequency of cancers in different familial phenotypes. J Med Genet 2010;47(6): 421–8.
41. Morioka T, Miyoshi-Imamura T, Blyth BJ, et al. Ionizing radiation, inflammation, and their interactions in colon carcinogenesis in Mlh1-deficient mice. Cancer Sci 2015;106(3):217–26.

Multiple Endocrine Neoplasia Type 1 Syndrome Pancreatic Neuroendocrine Tumor Genotype/Phenotype

Is There Any Advance on Predicting or Preventing?

Bhavishya Ramamoorthy, MD, Naris Nilubol, MD*

KEYWORDS

- Multiple endocrine neoplasia type 1 syndrome (MEN1)
- Pancreatic neuroendocrine tumor (PNET) • Menin • Genotype • Phenotype
- Epigenetic

KEY POINTS

- Multiple endocrine neoplasia type 1 syndrome (MEN1) is classically characterized by hyperparathyroidism, pituitary adenomas, and entero-pancreatic neuroendocrine tumors.
- Entero-pancreatic neuroendocrine tumors are the most common cause of death in patients with MEN1.
- Menin is a ubiquitous protein that associates with many other proteins that control cell signaling and proliferation, as well as proteins involved in the epigenetic regulation of gene expression.
- Genotype–phenotype associations have not been firmly established, but some studies indicate a correlation between mutations in exons 2, 9, and 10 and malignant pancreatic neuroendocrine tumors (PNETs) in MEN1 patients.
- Epigenetic studies have shown differences in DNA methylation between MEN1-associated PNETs and sporadic PNETs, but further investigation into DNA methylation, histone modification, and noncoding RNAs is needed to determine epigenetic–phenotypic associations.

Surgical Oncology Program, Endocrine Surgery Section, National Cancer Institute, NIH, 10 Center Drive, Building 10 – Room 45952, Bethesda, MD 20892, USA
* Corresponding author.
E-mail address: naris.nilubol@nih.gov

Surg Oncol Clin N Am 32 (2023) 315–325
https://doi.org/10.1016/j.soc.2022.10.008
1055-3207/23/Published by Elsevier Inc.

MULTIPLE ENDOCRINE NEOPLASIA TYPE 1 SYNDROME: PREVALENCE AND DIAGNOSIS

Multiple endocrine neoplasia type 1 syndrome (MEN1) is a rare autosomal dominant disease caused by inactivating mutations in the tumor suppressor gene *MEN1*, which predisposes patients to the development of characteristic endocrine and non-endocrine tumors.[1–7] Classically, MEN1 is associated with primary hyperparathyroidism from multiglandular hyperplastic parathyroid tumors, anterior pituitary adenomas, and entero-pancreatic neuroendocrine tumors.[3,7] Other tumors that have also been implicated in MEN1 include thymic, pulmonary, and gastric neuroendocrine tumors, adrenocortical tumors, (rarely) pheochromocytoma, central nervous system tumors including meningiomas, schwannomas, and ependymomas, and soft-tissue tumors such as lipomas, leiomyomas, angiofibromas, collagenomas, and hibernomas; more recently, female MEN1 patients have been found to have increased risk of breast cancer.[8]

Though rare, with a prevalence of 3 to 20 cases per 100,000 individuals, the disease shows high age-dependent penetrance; more than 50% of patients present with clinical features by age 20 years old, 95% by age 40,[1] and approximately 100% by age 50.[9] There is no observed ethnic or racial predisposition, but some studies have shown a slight female predominance.[1,9]

According to the Clinical Practice Guidelines, MEN1 can be diagnosed if patients meet clinical (two or more principal MEN1-associated tumors), familial (one MEN1-associated tumor and a first-degree relative with MEN1), or genetic criteria (MEN1 mutation without clinical or biochemical manifestations).[7] It is most commonly encountered as an inherited autosomal dominant disorder, as is the case in over 90% of cases; however, *de novo MEN1* mutations can occur (<10%), whereby a *MEN1* mutation develops in the embryo.[3,10,11] As described in Knudson's two-hit hypothesis for tumor suppressor genes, the germline inactivating mutation creates heterozygosity of the gene, but it is the second somatic inactivating mutation to the remaining allele that leads to loss of heterozygosity and the development of tumors and the clinical manifestations of the disease.

MULTIPLE ENDOCRINE NEOPLASIA TYPE 1 SYNDROME: MENIN

The *MEN1* tumor suppressor gene is located on chromosome 11q13.[1,3,5,12] The gene's 10 exons encode menin, a 610 amino acid, 67 kDa protein that is widely expressed and predominantly localizes to the nucleus, though some studies show some menin protein may associate with the cell membrane. Importantly, it contains three nuclear localization signals in the C-terminal region. The protein structurally encompasses a binding pocket that facilitates interactions with proteins such as

Table 1				
Pancreatic neuroendocrine neoplasm classifications				
PanNENs	**Differentiation**		**Proliferation Features**	
		Grade	**Ki67 (% per ≥500 cells)**	**Mitotic Count (per 10 HPF)**
PNET	Well differentiated	G1 (low)	<3	<2
		G2 (intermediate)	3–20	2 to 20
		G3 (high)	>20	>20
PNEC	Poorly differentiated	G3 (high)	>20	>20

transcription factors, histone modifiers, cytoskeletal proteins, and cytosolic cell signaling proteins.[1,5,13] Through inhibitory interactions with transcription factors JunD, the NFKB family, and the Smad family, and with activator of S-phase kinase (ASK), menin represses the activation of multiple pathways involved in cellular proliferation.[14] In addition, menin interacts with histone methyltransferase mixed-lineage leukemia complexes,[13–18] enabling methylation of the lysine 4 residue on histone H3; this trimethylation of H3K4 (H3K4me3) subsequently facilitates the transcriptional activation of cyclin-dependent kinase inhibitors p18 and p27, preventing unopposed cell-cycle progression. Its role in genome stability is implied through interactions with a subunit of replication protein A (RPA2) and FANCD2 protein, both of which are involved in DNA repair.[14] Menin also interacts directly with double-stranded DNA via its nuclear localization signals; it has been reported to cause upregulation of caspase 8 transcription and downregulation of insulin growth factor binding protein-2 (IGFBP-2) transcription. Further interactions and effects exist but have not been fully elucidated yet. Overall, menin has been shown to play a key regulatory role in cell cycle progression and proliferation.

MULTIPLE ENDOCRINE NEOPLASIA TYPE 1 SYNDROME: CLINICAL MANIFESTATIONS

As stated previously, the principal MEN1 clinical manifestations are primary hyperparathyroidism, pituitary adenomas, and entero-pancreatic neuroendocrine tumors, which develop in 90%, 30 to 40%, and 30 to 70% of patients, respectively, by age 40.[3,7] Primary hyperparathyroidism is seen in 100% of patients by age 50 and is the most common first manifestation of the disease (90%).[4,6] Important differences exist between sporadic hyperparathyroidism and hyperparathyroidism secondary to MEN1. Unlike patients with sporadic primary hyperparathyroidism, patients with MEN1 commonly present at a younger age with no female gender predilection, in concordance with an autosomal dominant inheritance pattern.[3,9] In addition, though patients with MEN1 tend to have lower calcium and PTH levels, the severity of bone mineral loss and nephrolithiasis is higher compared with sporadic hyperparathyroidism, and hyperparathyroidism associated with MEN1 is caused by multiple parathyroid gland hyperplasia rather than a solitary parathyroid adenoma,[3,9] although asymmetric hyperplasia can give the appearance of adenomas. In the setting of Zollinger–Ellison syndrome (ZES) caused by gastrinomas, which is the most common functional PNET in MEN1, the correction of hypercalcemia with parathyroidectomy has been shown to reduce gastrin secretion and acid output.[19]

Anterior pituitary tumors are identified in approximately 30% to 40% of patients with MEN1, and although approximately two-thirds of patients have microadenomas, the rates of macroadenomas are higher in patients with MEN1 than in patients without the syndrome.[1,9] Prolactinomas are by far the most commonly encountered pituitary tumor in MEN1, with a prevalence of 65%, followed by somatotropinomas, ACTH-producing adenomas, and gonadotropin-producing adenomas; interestingly, adenomas secreting multiple hormones have been seen in up to 10% of MEN1-associated pituitary adenomas.[9] Of note, there is a documented familial MEN1 variant called the Burin variant with a high rate of prolactinomas but a low rate of entero-pancreatic neuroendocrine tumors, particularly gastrinomas that were seen in only 10% of the patient group.[20]

Entero-pancreatic neuroendocrine tumors are seen in 70% to 80% of patients with MEN1 and carry significant clinical importance as they are the most common cause of death in patients with MEN1 due to the risk of metastasis.[6,9] Most commonly observed are nonfunctional neuroendocrine tumors, which are seen in 55% of patients with

MEN1; these carry a higher mortality rate than functional tumors, likely as a result of delayed diagnosis in the absence of clinical symptoms caused by abnormal hormone secretion. Of note, this group encompasses tumors that truly do not secrete hormones, tumors that secrete hormones at levels insufficient to cause a clinical syndrome, and tumors that secrete hormones that do not cause a clinical syndrome. The most common functional entero-pancreatic neuroendocrine tumor is gastrinomas, which are associated with ZES. Interestingly, they are not the most prevalent PNET in MEN1 patients and are, in fact, encountered as duodenal microtumors in 80% of MEN1-associated gastrinoma cases. Others include insulinomas, glucagonomas, VIPomas, and somatostatinomas. These will be discussed in greater detail in a later section of the review.

PANCREATIC NEUROENDOCRINE TUMORS

Pancreatic neuroendocrine neoplasms (PanNENs) are composed of cancer cells that express both neuroendocrine markers (eg, chromogranin A and synaptophysin) and pancreatic tissue-specific markers; this subset of tumors has undergone multiple classification changes over the last two decades by the World Health Organization (WHO), most recently in 2017.[21] Currently, PanNENs are divided into well-differentiated PNETs and poorly differentiated pancreatic neuroendocrine carcinomas (PNECs). PNECs by definition have morphology demonstrating poor differentiation and high-grade (G3) proliferation criteria, that is, Ki67 staining index of >20% of $\geq$500 cells and mitotic count of >20 per 10 high-powered fields (HPF). In contrast, PNETs are subdivided into low-grade (G1), intermediate-grade (G2), and high-grade (G3) again based on proliferation markers Ki67 and mitotic index; this allows for the classification of a subset of PanNENs that are both well-differentiated and with high proliferation indices **Table 1**.

PNETs account for less than 3% of pancreatic neoplasms in the general population, with an incidence of 0.8 cases per 100,000 persons.[17,22–24] Only 5% to 10% arise in the setting of predisposing genetic syndromes, which include MEN1, von Hippel Lindau syndrome (VHL), tuberous sclerosis complex (TSC), and neurofibromatosis type 1 (NF1).

In the general population, 15% of PNETs are functional and 85% are nonfunctional.[17] Functional PNETs are defined by the development of clinical symptoms rather than immunohistochemical findings, and nonfunctional PNETs are clinically silent, not necessarily nonsecretory. Nonfunctional PNETs carry a poorer prognosis, with 5-year survival rate of 30% to 40%, and are often not identified until their growth causes obstructive or compressive symptoms, at which point lymph node and liver metastases may be seen. Compared with sporadic PNETs, MEN1-associated PNETs are diagnosed at a younger age. In MEN1, PNETs have become more frequently identified and are now seen in up to 80% of patients, owing to increased and more effective surveillance strategies and modalities. Nonfunctional PNETs in the context of MEN1 are also most common (55% of cases), followed by insulinomas (7% to 31% of cases), and gastrinomas (5% of cases); glucagonomas (3% to 4% of cases), VIPomas (2% of cases), and somatostatinomas (2% of cases) are rare. Like the duodenal microgastrinomas commonly seen with MEN1-associated ZES, PNETs in MEN1 are much more commonly seen as multiple microadenomas (<0.5 cm).[3,17] Solitary PNETs in MEN1 patients, which occur less than 13% of the time, are usually >2 cm in size and nonfunctional.

The multifocal nature and genetic predisposition for the recurrence of MEN1-associated PNETs hold important implications for their treatment.[17,25] Currently, guidelines recommend observation for asymptomatic, nonfunctional PNETs that are less than 1 to 2 cm with surveillance imaging every 6 to 12 months to monitor size changes.[23,26,27] Increased tumor size correlates with metastases and intermediate or high grade with higher recurrence rate.[23,27] Because these tumors are often identified in young patients with multiple small tumors, complete surgical resection may entail major pancreatic resection with risks of pancreatic exocrine insufficiency and diabetes. Management of functional PNETs depends on tumor type and symptom.[3] Gastrinomas, which are most often seen in MEN1 as multiple microadenomas in the duodenum, are typically managed medically with proton pump inhibitors, histamine receptor blockers, and somatostatin analogs to control the effects of excess gastrin. At the time of diagnosis, gastrinomas are seen with lymph node metastases in 34% to 85% and liver metastases in 6% to 16% of cases. Surgical resection is indicated in cases with concomitant nonfunctional PNET that meets resection criteria (eg, >2 cm in size or doubles in size in 6 months). In contrast to gastrinomas, insulinomas are found as solitary tumors in 85%, multiple in 6% to 13%, and with other PNETs in 10% of cases. Although the tumors are usually small (<2 cm) and metastatic disease is uncommon (4% to 14% of cases), medical management is typically unsuccessful in curtailing hyperinsulinism symptoms. The tumors are found in the equal distribution in all regions of the pancreas, and surgical resection is indicated if the tumor(s) can be localized, as these PNETs can often be completely resected and achieve surgical cure without an extensive pancreatic resection, though the risk of recurrence remains. Glucagonomas and VIPomas are characteristically found in the body and tail of the pancreas. Glucagonomas are associated with necrolytic migratory erythema, weight loss, anemia, and stomatitis, and there is a 50% to 80% rate of metastatic disease at the time of diagnosis. VIPomas present with the classic triad of watery diarrhea, hypokalemia, and achlorydia. Metastasis is common in patients with glucagonoma and VIPoma. Like insulinomas, both glucagonomas and VIPomas should be resected if localized.

GENOTYPE–PHENOTYPE CORRELATIONS IN MULTIPLE ENDOCRINE NEOPLASIA TYPE 1 SYNDROME-ASSOCIATED PANCREATIC NEUROENDOCRINE TUMORS

Because entero-pancreatic neuroendocrine tumors are the most common cause of death in patients with MEN1 due to the risk of metastatic disease,[6,9] it would be beneficial to identify prognostic factors that could help identify patients with MEN1 that may benefit for more aggressive screening, surveillance, and treatment of PNETs. For this reason, many studies have been performed in an attempt to establish genotype–phenotype correlations. However, unlike the accurate genotype–phenotype correlation seen in APC and RET, that of MEN1 remains unclear, partly due to the complex functions of menin, including epigenetic regulation of gene expression.

One of the first investigations by Bartsch and colleagues[28] identified 21 patients with MEN1 and pancreaticoduodenal neuroendocrine tumors who had 14 different mutations and found that those with truncating nonsense mutations and frameshift mutations involving exons 2, 9, and 10, which comprise the N- and C-terminal regions, had significantly higher rates of malignant tumors, 55% compared with 10%. Other studies have found that MEN1 mutations in exons 2, 9, and 10 are the most common mutations seen in patients with MEN1-associated gastroenteropancreatic neuroendocrine tumors (GEP-NETs), but some studies show higher rates of frameshift mutations,[29] and others show higher rates of nonsense mutations.[4] Kövesdi and colleagues[30] corroborated the finding of high frequency of frameshift and nonsense mutations in MEN-1-associated GEP-NETs, identifying a significantly higher rate of high-impact mutations, defined as frameshift mutations, nonsense mutations, a splice-site mutation, and a large deletion, compared with low-impact mutations, defined as missense mutations and in-frame deletions.

Christakis and colleagues[31] found that MEN1 patients with PNETs were more likely to have a mutation in exon 2 than in any other exon and more likely to have a frameshift mutation. Deleterious exon 2 mutations were significantly more likely to be associated with malignant PNET and with distant metastasis from a PNET than deleterious mutations in exons 3 to 10, and they trended toward shorter overall survival.

In a comparison between hereditary and sporadic PNETs, one study with 58 patients with MEN1 found a strong negative correlation between frameshift or splice-site mutations and stage.[24] They also found that exon 5 mutations were diagnosed with PNETs at an earlier age than mutations in other locations, and they found that exon 2 mutations were associated with more frequent metastases.

Contrastingly, a study by Bartsch and colleagues[32] did not identify any genotype–phenotype differences between the 36 truncating and 9 nontruncating MEN1 mutations in their cohort of 71 patients. They did, however, compare mutations affecting menin protein's interacting domains with JunD, Smad3, CHES1, and HDAC1 and found that mutations causing loss of interaction (LOI) with CHES1, which are encompassed in exons 9 and 10, were associated with significantly higher rates of functional PNETs, malignant PNETs, PNETs with distant metastasis, and PNET-related deaths. Another study by Thevenon and colleagues[33] examined 262 mutations in 806 MEN1 patients and found no genotype–phenotype correlations regarding PNETs but did identify an increased risk of overall MEN1-related death in mutations that caused LOI with JunD.

In sum, genotype–phenotype correlations have yet to be firmly established in MEN1 PNETs. However, certain trends, such as truncating or deleterious mutations in exons 2, 9, and 10 have been documented in multiple studies (**Table 2**).

EPIGENETIC MECHANISMS IN MULTIPLE ENDOCRINE NEOPLASIA TYPE 1 SYNDROME-ASSOCIATED PANCREATIC NEUROENDOCRINE TUMORS

Although genotype–phenotype correlations in MEN1 PNETs have not been consistently shown, other studies have begun exploring the impact of epigenetic changes on MEN1-associated PNETs and have yielded interesting results. DNA methylation is a well-documented epigenetic mechanism of gene expression silencing.[15,34] Methylation of CpG DNA sites in promoter regions is accomplished by DNA methyltransferase enzymes (DNMTs), and hypermethylation of tumor suppressor genes' promoter regions is often seen in the setting of cancer. In sporadic PNETs, the Ras-association domain gene family 1 (RASSF1) tumor suppressor gene promoter is the most commonly hypermethylated promoter region, seen in 75% to 83% of sporadic PNETs. Hypermethylation of the RASSF1 promoter is more frequently identified in metastatic PNETs than nonmetastatic PNETs, implying a role in neuroendocrine tumor progression. Other hypermethylated genes have been implicated in sporadic PNETs but differentially depending on functional type; for example, CDKN2A/p16INK4a promoter hypermethylation and IGF2 hypomethylation have been associated with gastrinomas.[15] IGF2 hypermethylation is commonly identified in insulinomas, whereas CDKN2A/p16INK4a alterations are uncommon.[15]

MEN1-associated PNETs also show hypermethylation of tumor suppressor genes but in different patterns than in sporadic PNETs. Conemans and colleagues[35] showed no difference in cumulative methylation index (CMI) between MEN1-associated PNETs and sporadic PNETs, but hypermethylation of CASP8, RASSF1_1, and RASSF1_2 were identified more often in MEN1-associated PNETs than sporadic

Table 2
Summary of *MEN1* mutation characteristics in pancreatic neuroendocrine tumors

Study, Year	Mutation Type	Exon	Association
Bartsch et al.[28] 2000	Truncating frameshift or nonsense	2, 9, and 10	Increased risk of malignant PNET
Thevenon et al.[33] 2013	Loss of interaction with JunD		Increased overall risk of MEN1-related death
Bartsch et al.[32] 2014	Loss of interaction with CHES1	9 and 10	Increased risk of functional PNET, malignant PNET, PNET with metastasis, and PNET-related death
Christakis et al. 2017	Deleterious	2	Increased risk of malignant PNET and PNET with metastasis
Marini et al. 2018	Frameshift	2, 9, and 10	GEP-NET
Marini et al. 2018	Nonsense	2, 9, and 10	GEP-NET
Kövesdi et al.[30] 2019	Frameshift, nonsense, splice-site, large deletion		GEP-NET
Soczomski et al.[24] 2021		5 2	Earlier age of PNET diagnosis Increased risk of PNET with metastasis

PNETs. MEN1 subgroup analyses revealed that nonfunctional MEN1-associated PNETs had higher CMI if they were >2 cm or had liver metastases and that MEN1 insulinomas more frequently had hypermethylation of *RASSF1_1* than nonfunctional PNETs (70% vs 47%), whereas nonfunctional PNETs more frequently had hypermethylation of *MGMT2* than insulinomas (44.7% vs 8.3%). Another study by Tirosh and colleagues[36] included 96 NETS, of which 42 were from MEN1 patients and 24 were specifically MEN1-associated PNETs, and also showed MEN1-associated NETs and sporadic NETs had similar percentages of hypermethylated regions. However, they identified different methylation profiles associated with NET location and found higher percentages of *APC* promoter hypermethylation in MEN1-associated NETs compared with sporadic NETs, though these were more often seen in gastric and duodenal NETs compared with small intestine NETs and PNETs. A smaller investigation focusing on nonfunctional PNETs compared nine sporadic, ten MEN1-associated, and ten VHL-associated tumors and found that MEN1-associated nonfunctional PNETs had significantly more hypermethylated genomic regions compared with the others, the majority of which were associated with downregulation of gene expression[37]; some of these downregulated genes include *RBM47*, *FAM3B*, *ECHDC1*, *MPP2*, *JAK1*, *ATP11A*, and *CDCA7L*. Of these, *RBM47* and *CDCA7L* are associated with other cancer types, *RBM47* with colorectal, breast, and lung cancer and *CDCA7L* with hepatocellular carcinoma. Subsequently activated pathways for MEN1-associated nonfunctional PNETs included VEGF signaling, neuronal pathways, insulin secretion regulation, and the phosphatidylinositol-4,5-bisphosphate (PIP2) related pathway. By contrast, VHL-associated nonfunctional PNETs were more frequently associated with hypomethylation and activation of pathways involved in VEGF and beta cell development.

Chromatin remodeling via histone modifications is another epigenetic avenue under investigation. As stated previously, menin interacts with histone methyltransferase MLL complexes, facilitating trimethylation of H3K4 (H3K4me3), an activating epigenetic marker. *Men1* knockout mouse models have shown a cooperative effect between MLL and menin where inactivation of MLL1, also known as KMT2A, in *Men1* knockout mice have reduced survival, and their pancreata show accelerated pancreatic islet tumor progression with tumors that were more frequently larger, more vascular, and more cellularly abnormal.[38] Another study using *Men1* knockout mice pancreata showed decreased islet tumorigenesis and prolonged survival with inactivation of retinoblastoma binding protein 2 (RBP2), an H3K4me3 demethylase,[39] suggesting that RBP2 is a downstream effector of menin. One interesting study further showed this by showing that the deletion of RBP2 leads to a reversal in the downregulation of IGFBP2 in MEN1-deficient islets.[40]

MicroRNAs (miRNAs) are a class of small noncoding RNAs that downregulate or silence gene expression through.[12,18] Some studies have examined miRNA expression profiles in PNET patients, and although some intriguing results have revealed differential expression profiles in different types of GEP-NETs by location and identified miR-21 as a miRNA significantly upregulated in metastatic PNETs, none of these studies specifically examine MEN1-associated PNETs.[12]

FUTURE DIRECTIONS

Genotype–phenotype correlations in MEN1-associated PNETs remain an area of investigation. As a major cause of morbidity and mortality in patients with MEN1, identifying these correlations may assist in the screening, surveillance, and treatment recommendations for patients based on their genotypes. However, despite several attempts to identify clear associations, none have been firmly established, though trends have emerged. MEN1 patients with PNETs and deleterious mutations in exons 2, 9, and 10 may benefit from closer follow-up and surveillance, and perhaps more aggressive treatment.

Exploration into epigenetic factors has yielded interesting and promising early data. As this field expands and more investigations are performed with a specific focus on MEN1-associated PNETs, it is possible that new relationships will be identified. In addition, as epigenetic changes are reversible, medications that target epigenetic regulatory modifications may become of interest. For example, azacitidine and decitabine, both of which are DNA methyltransferase inhibitors, are approved for the treatment of myelodysplastic syndrome.[39] Further investigation is needed to verify and elucidate the underlying causes of genotype–phenotype and epigenetic–phenotypic correlations that have been suggested.

SUMMARY

One of the most common manifestations of MEN1 is PNET. Compared with sporadic PNETs, MEN1-associated PNETs tend to be multifocal with high rates of recurrence, often making complete surgical resection difficult or involving major organ resection. *MEN1* mutations in exons 2, 9, and 10 may be associated with increased risk for malignant PNETs, but clear genotype–phenotype correlations have yet to be validated. Further study into menin's role in gene expression through epigenetic modifications may provide additional clues to detect patients with MEN1-associated PNETs that are at greater risk of aggressive disease who subsequently may benefit from closer follow-up and treatment.

ACKNOWLEDGMENTS

The research activity in this article was supported by the National Institutes of Health Intramural Research Program (# ZIA BC 011286).

CONFLICT OF INTERESTS

The authors declare no conflict of interest.

REFERENCES

1. Brandi ML, Agarwal SK, Perrier ND, et al. Multiple Endocrine Neoplasia Type 1: Latest Insights. Endocr Rev 2021;42(2):133–70.
2. de Laat JM, van der Luijt RB, Pieterman CR, et al. MEN1 redefined, a clinical comparison of mutation-positive and mutation-negative patients. BMC Med 2016;14(1):182.
3. Kamilaris CDC, Stratakis CA. Multiple Endocrine Neoplasia Type 1 (MEN1): An Update and the Significance of Early Genetic and Clinical Diagnosis. Front Endocrinol (Lausanne) 2019;10:339.
4. Marini F, Giusti F, Fossi C, et al. Multiple endocrine neoplasia type 1: analysis of germline MEN1 mutations in the Italian multicenter MEN1 patient database. Endocrine 2018;62(1):215–33, published correction appears in Endocrine. 2018 Jul 21.
5. Falchetti A. Genetics of multiple endocrine neoplasia type 1 syndrome: what's new and what's old. F1000Res 2017;6:F1000. Faculty Rev-73. Published 2017 Jan 24.
6. Mele C, Mencarelli M, Caputo M, et al. Phenotypes Associated With MEN1 Syndrome: A Focus on Genotype–phenotype Correlations. Front Endocrinol (Lausanne) 2020;11:591501.
7. Thakker RV, Newey PJ, Walls GV, et al. Clinical practice guidelines for multiple endocrine neoplasia type 1 (MEN1). J Clin Endocrinol Metab 2012;97(9): 2990–3011.
8. van Leeuwaarde RS, Dreijerink KM, Ausems MG, et al. MEN1-Dependent Breast Cancer: Indication for Early Screening? Results From the Dutch MEN1 Study Group. J Clin Endocrinol Metab 2017;102(6):2083–90.
9. Al-Salameh A, Cadiot G, Calender A, et al. Clinical aspects of multiple endocrine neoplasia type 1. Nat Rev Endocrinol 2021;17(4):207–24.
10. Giusti F, Cianferotti L, Boaretto F, et al. Multiple endocrine neoplasia syndrome type 1: institution, management, and data analysis of a nationwide multicenter patient database. Endocrine 2017;58(2):349–59.
11. Marini F, Carbonell Sala S, Falchetti A, et al. The genetic ascertainment of multiple endocrine neoplasia type 1 syndrome by ancient DNA analysis. J Endocrinol Invest 2008;31(10):905–9.
12. Donati S, Ciuffi S, Marini F, et al. Multiple Endocrine Neoplasia Type 1: The Potential Role of microRNAs in the Management of the Syndrome. Int J Mol Sci 2020; 21(20):7592.
13. Lips CJ, Dreijerink KM, Höppener JW. Variable clinical expression in patients with a germline MEN1 disease gene mutation: clues to a genotype–phenotype correlation. Clinics (Sao Paulo) 2012;67(Suppl 1):49–56.
14. Lemos MC, Thakker RV. Multiple endocrine neoplasia type 1 (MEN1): analysis of 1336 mutations reported in the first decade following identification of the gene. Hum Mutat 2008;29(1):22–32.
15. Karpathakis A, Dibra H, Thirlwell C. Neuroendocrine tumours: cracking the epigenetic code. Endocr Relat Cancer 2013;20(3):R65–82.
16. Pipinikas CP, Berner AM, Sposito T, et al. The evolving (epi)genetic landscape of pancreatic neuroendocrine tumours. Endocr Relat Cancer 2019;26(9):R519–44.

17. Marini F, Giusti F, Tonelli F, et al. Pancreatic Neuroendocrine Neoplasms in Multiple Endocrine Neoplasia Type 1. Int J Mol Sci 2021;22(8):4041.

18. Iyer S, Agarwal SK. Epigenetic regulation in the tumorigenesis of MEN1-associated endocrine cell types. J Mol Endocrinol 2018;61(1):R13–24.

19. Norton JA, Venzon DJ, Berna MJ, et al. Prospective study of surgery for primary hyperparathyroidism (HPT) in multiple endocrine neoplasia-type 1 and Zollinger-Ellison syndrome: long-term outcome of a more virulent form of HPT. Ann Surg 2008;247(3):501–10.

20. Hao W, Skarulis MC, Simonds WF, et al. Multiple endocrine neoplasia type 1 variant with frequent prolactinoma and rare gastrinoma. J Clin Endocrinol Metab 2004;89(8):3776–84.

21. Inzani F, Petrone G, Rindi G. The New World Health Organization Classification for Pancreatic Neuroendocrine Neoplasia. Endocrinol Metab Clin North Am 2018; 47(3):463–70.

22. Partelli S, Giannone F, Schiavo Lena M, et al. Is the Real Prevalence of Pancreatic Neuroendocrine Tumors Underestimated? A Retrospective Study on a Large Series of Pancreatic Specimens. Neuroendocrinology 2019;109(2):165–70.

23. Howe JR, Merchant NB, Conrad C, et al. The North American Neuroendocrine Tumor Society Consensus Paper on the Surgical Management of Pancreatic Neuroendocrine Tumors. Pancreas 2020;49(1):1–33.

24. Soczomski P, Jurecka-Lubieniecka B, Krzywon A, et al. A Direct Comparison of Patients With Hereditary and Sporadic Pancreatic Neuroendocrine Tumors: Evaluation of Clinical Course, Prognostic Factors and Genotype–phenotype Correlations. Front Endocrinol (Lausanne) 2021;12:681013.

25. Jensen RT, Norton JA. Treatment of Pancreatic Neuroendocrine Tumors in Multiple Endocrine Neoplasia Type 1: Some Clarity But Continued Controversy. Pancreas 2017;46(5):589–94.

26. Niederle B, Selberherr A, Bartsch DK, et al. Multiple Endocrine Neoplasia Type 1 and the Pancreas: Diagnosis and Treatment of Functioning and Non-Functioning Pancreatic and Duodenal Neuroendocrine Neoplasia within the MEN1 Syndrome - An International Consensus Statement. Neuroendocrinology 2021;111(7): 609–30.

27. Sadowski SM, Pieterman CRC, Perrier ND, et al. Prognostic factors for the outcome of nonfunctioning pancreatic neuroendocrine tumors in MEN1: a systematic review of literature. Endocr Relat Cancer 2020;27(6):R145–61.

28. Bartsch DK, Langer P, Wild A, et al. Pancreaticoduodenal endocrine tumors in multiple endocrine neoplasia type 1: surgery or surveillance? Surgery 2000; 128(6):958–66.

29. Marini F, Giusti F, Brandi ML. Multiple endocrine neoplasia type 1: extensive analysis of a large database of Florentine patients. Orphanet J Rare Dis 2018; 13(1):205.

30. Kövesdi A, Tóth M, Butz H, et al. True MEN1 or phenocopy? Evidence for genophenotypic correlations in MEN1 syndrome. Endocrine 2019;65(2):451–9.

31. Christakis I, Qiu W, Hyde SM, et al. Genotype–phenotype pancreatic neuroendocrine tumor relationship in multiple endocrine neoplasia type 1 patients: A 23-year experience at a single institution. Surgery 2018;163(1):212–7.

32. Bartsch DK, Slater EP, Albers M, et al. Higher risk of aggressive pancreatic neuroendocrine tumors in MEN1 patients with MEN1 mutations affecting the CHES1 interacting MENIN domain. J Clin Endocrinol Metab 2014;99(11):E2387–91.

33. Thevenon J, Bourredjem A, Faivre L, et al. Higher risk of death among MEN1 patients with mutations in the JunD interacting domain: a Groupe d'etude des Tumeurs Endocrines (GTE) cohort study. Hum Mol Genet 2013;22(10):1940–8.
34. Tirosh A, Kebebew E. Genetic and epigenetic alterations in pancreatic neuroendocrine tumors. J Gastrointest Oncol 2020;11(3):567–77.
35. Conemans EB, Lodewijk L, Moelans CB, et al. DNA methylation profiling in MEN1-related pancreatic neuroendocrine tumors reveals a potential epigenetic target for treatment. Eur J Endocrinol 2018;179(3):153–60.
36. Tirosh A, Killian JK, Petersen D, et al. Distinct DNA Methylation Signatures in Neuroendocrine Tumors Specific for Primary Site and Inherited Predisposition. J Clin Endocrinol Metab 2020;105(10):3285–94.
37. Tirosh A, Mukherjee S, Lack J, et al. Distinct genome-wide methylation patterns in sporadic and hereditary nonfunctioning pancreatic neuroendocrine tumors. Cancer 2019;125(8):1247–57.
38. Lin W, Francis JM, Li H, et al. Kmt2a cooperates with menin to suppress tumorigenesis in mouse pancreatic islets. Cancer Biol Ther 2016;17(12):1274–81.
39. Lin W, Cao J, Liu J, et al. Loss of the retinoblastoma binding protein 2 (RBP2) histone demethylase suppresses tumorigenesis in mice lacking Rb1 or Men1. Proc Natl Acad Sci U S A 2011;108(33):13379–86.
40. Lin W, Watanabe H, Peng S, et al. Dynamic epigenetic regulation by menin during pancreatic islet tumor formation. Mol Cancer Res 2015;13(4):689–98.

Minimally Invasive Pancreatectomy
Robotic and Laparoscopic Developments

Seth J. Concors, MD, Matthew H.G. Katz, MD,
Naruhiko Ikoma, MD, MS*

KEYWORDS

- Pancreatectomy • Minimally invasive surgery • Surgery • Robotic • Laparoscopy
- Pancreatic neuroendocrine tumor

KEY POINTS

- Minimally invasive pancreatectomy has increased in utilization, with widespread adoption of robotic surgery.
- When preformed at high-volume centers by expert surgeons, minimally invasive pancreatectomy has been associated with shorter hospital stay, less blood loss, and equivalent complication rates compared with open pancreatectomy.
- The primary challenge to adoption of minimally invasive techniques in pancreatectomy beyond expert centers is the maintenance high-quality oncologic surgical standards.

Abbreviations	
SMV	superior mesenteric vein
PV	portal vein
NCDB	National Cancer Database
HJ	hepaticojejunostomy
PJ	pancreatojejunostomy
PDS	polydioxanone

INTRODUCTION

Minimally invasive techniques have been increasingly used in oncologic surgery and pancreatic surgery in particular.[1–6] Minimally invasive pancreatectomy (MIP) has been performed with increasing frequency in all pancreatic pathologies, including pancreatic neuroendocrine tumors (PNETs), including pancreaticoduodenectomy (PD), distal pancreatectomy (DP), and pancreatic enucleation.[7–9]

Department of Surgical Oncology, The University of Texas MD Anderson Cancer Center, 1400 Pressler, FCT 17.6022, Houston, TX 77030, USA
* Corresponding author.
E-mail address: nikoma@mdanderson.org
Twitter: @SethConcorsMD (S.J.C.); @MKatzMD (M.H.G.K.); @IkomaMD (N.I.)

Surg Oncol Clin N Am 32 (2023) 327–342
https://doi.org/10.1016/j.soc.2022.10.009
1055-3207/23/© 2022 Elsevier Inc. All rights reserved.
surgonc.theclinics.com

Robotic-assisted surgery using the *DaVinci* platform has accelerated the adoption of MIP. The proportion of robotic DP between 2015 and 2016 was nearly 4 times greater than between 2010 and -2012 (16% vs 4%), with a similar increase in proportion of robotic PD (7% vs 2%) over the same time frame.[1] Advantages of robotic surgery over laparoscopy include three-dimensional visualization, increased degrees of motion with endo-articulation, stable camera platform, surgeon ergonomics, and single surgeon's ability to control four instruments. Systematic adoption of MIP has been facilitated by the creation of multiple multicenter training programs in robotic DP and PD, aiming to standardize the oncologic safety and technical performance of these operations.[10–12]

Maintaining the quality of oncologic pancreatectomy with continued uptake of minimally invasive surgery remains the most critical challenge going forward. Variation in surgical quality directly impacts locoregional recurrence and long-term survival in patients with colorectal cancer.[13] In pancreatic cancer, obtaining a margin-negative resection is an independent predictor of survival.[14] In PD, complete clearance of the lateral aspect of the superior mesenteric artery (SMA) is critical in improving chances of R0 resection.[14,15] Whether surgeons beginning to adapt MIP will be able to sustain these technical requirements are paramount to broader success of this approach. Given these concerns, the US Food and Drug Administration has cautioned against the use of robotic-assisted surgery for oncologic indications, given a lack of evidence demonstrating equivalent overall survival and oncologic outcomes.[16]

Evidence supporting the association between MIP and decreased length of stay, lower blood loss, and equivalent complication rates has largely been reported at high-volume centers with experienced surgeons.[17–19] The Miami Guidelines for Minimally Invasive Pancreas Resection recommended minimally invasive DP in experienced hands for benign or low-grade malignant tumors suggest it is an equivalent approach in pancreas ductal adenocarcinoma and that insufficient data exist to recommend minimally invasive PD.[20] These international expert guidelines note that randomized controlled studies are needed for both DP and PD.

Here, we review the existing literature in MIP and describe the technical approach of the most commonly performed procedures for PNETs: DP, PD, and pancreatic enucleation. As we perform robotic-assisted surgery, they describe technical considerations to this approach, with similar techniques applicable to laparoscopic surgery.

General Indications and Patient Selection

Perioperative multidisciplinary planning is the key to success of both open and MIP. Perioperative assessment of cardiovascular, nutritional, and functional status is paramount to both short- and long-term outcomes after pancreatectomy, regardless of approach. Evidence continues to accumulate demonstrating the added value of nutritional evaluation and prehabilitation before pancreatectomy to enhance postoperative functional recovery.[21,22] In addition, in our experience, consistent operating room teams including nursing staff, surgical technicians, and anesthesiologists for MIP ensures the safest possible perioperative course.

Although the indications for MIP are the same to the open approach, careful case selection for MIP ensures adequate safety and success especially early in the learning curve. No randomized controlled data exist to guide patient selection, and one recent survey across Europe demonstrated that patient selection was largely driven by personal experience, rather than data.[23] We believe that evaluation of patient and surgical factors is critical in selecting the appropriate cases for MIP.

Patient factors

1. Patients at the extremes of body mass index (BMI) may pose technical challenges for both robotic and laparoscopic approaches. BMI has not shown to be associated with increased perioperative complications, particularly after minimally invasive DP, but may present added technical challenge in manipulation of the colonic mesentery and mobilization of the proximal jejunum.[24,25] Indeed, internal adiposity rather than BMI itself is more of problem in MIS approach. Particularly in robotic approach, subcutaneous fat and abdominal thickness has small impact on surgical difficulty.[26] Preoperative exercise program with weight reduction diet would make the operation safer in morbidly obese patients by reducing internal obesity and creating more surgical space with pneumoperitoneum.[27] In low BMI patients, adequate port spacing and intrabdominal surgical working room may present a challenge.
2. Prior history of pancreatitis, metallic biliary stent placement, and receipt of radiation therapy anecdotally increases difficulty of MIP due to desmoplastic changes surrounding pancreas and vascular structures, although severity of such desmoplastic change is difficult to expect before surgery. If radiographically evident pancreatitis is seen, waiting for 8 to 12 weeks before attempting resection is encouraged. After administration of radiation therapy, it is recommended to wait less than 12 weeks before attempting MIP.
3. Prior surgery history may increase complexity and operative time due to potentially lengthy lysis of adhesions. Particularly early in the learning curve when MIP has increased operative length, the addition of extended adhesiolysis is not recommended. Prior Roux-en-Y gastric bypass additionally adds complexity to operative conduct during minimally invasive PD.
4. Severe cardiopulmonary disease limiting pneumoperitoneum is a contraindication. Risks and benefits of MIS approach should be carefully considered for patients with marginal renal function (CKD 3) as pneumoperitoneum reduces venous return and may affect renal arterial flow.

Surgical factors

1. The need for multi-visceral or major vascular resection should represent a relative contraindication to MIP, especially early in the procedural learning curve. Although the robotic approach is technically feasible for vascular reconstruction, the lack of "surgeon's left hand" to control bleeding when it is needed is critical concern for safety in MIP. Zureikat and colleagues[18] demonstrated unchanged perioperative outcomes with increasingly complex R-PD, involving vascular resection, over the first 500 cases at their institution. Although these types of resections are not contraindications at highly experienced centers, they should be undertaken with caution. Tumors which require resection of the portal or superior mesenteric vein should be approached open outside of highly selected centers in highly selected circumstances.
2. A thorough review of high-quality CT scan with arterial and portal venous phases is critical in planning of operative approach for MIP. Replaced or aberrant vascular anatomy should be identified and taken into account in selecting patients for MIP. Replaced right hepatic artery while increasing the complexity of resection is not an absolute contraindication unless involved in the tumor process.[28]
3. For surgeons at the beginning of their learning curve selection of cases with imaging suggestive of dilated pancreatic and bile ducts facilitates ease of reconstruction and may minimize the risk of postoperative pancreatic or biliary fistulas.

Learning Curve

Volume-outcome relationships in gastrointestinal surgery, including pancreatic surgery, have been widely studied.[29,30] Although the case volumes of specific surgeries have been reported as meaningful in overcoming the learning curve of a new procedure, it is intuitive that experience with similarly complex foregut gastrointestinal procedures can accelerate the mastery of a similar procedure. In the Netherlands, Busweiler and colleagues[31] reported that the composite volume of gastric, esophageal, and pancreatic cancer resections at a given institution correlated with improvements in oncologic outcomes as well as overall survival after surgery for gastric cancer.

One of the largest obstacles to implementation of an MIP program is the learning curve, particularly in PD. As surgeons have been performing laparoscopic surgery for far long, more data exist for the learning curve in laparoscopic PD. This previous work has demonstrated three phases in development of technical proficiency in laparoscopic PD: the initial learning period, technical competence, and challenging period—with step-wise decreases in blood loss, length of stay, and operative time and increases in lymph node harvest.[32] A wide variety of case volume has been reported as necessary for overcoming the learning curve in laparoscopic PD, from 10 to 60 cases, with most authors suggesting around 60 to 80 cases.[32–34] Similarly, the learning curve needed to produce proficiency in robotic PD has been reported around 80 cases, with early optimization of blood loss and conversion to open around 20 cases, decreased rates of pancreatic fistula (POPF) and operative time after 40 and 80 cases, respectively.[35] The surgical group at the University of Pittsburgh has developed a robotic pancreatectomy program optimized to overcome this lengthy learning curve, with robust simulation and shared operative responsibilities.[36–39]

Minimally invasive DP follows a similar, though shorter, learning curve. In a recent meta-analysis Chan and colleagues[40] demonstrated both laparoscopic and robotic DP have a similar learning curve of 25.3 versus 20.7 cases respectively ($P = 0.6$) using a composite learning curve metric. The Pittsburgh group has reported 40 cases needed for optimization of robotic DP, with precipitous decrease in operative time between the first 20 and 40 cases (266 min and 210 min, respectively) and readmissions.[41]

In our robotic foregut surgery program, to accelerate the learning curve, we've developed a strategic approach to concentrating robotic foregut experience including pancreatectomy and gastrectomy and gradual increases in case complexity. Importantly, at our institution, we are prospectively monitoring outcomes of robotic foregut surgery under a protocol approved by the institutional review board. We initiated very early experience with cholecystectomy and gastrojejunostomy to get familiarized with robotic surgery platform and techniques of dissection and anastomosis. We performed progressively more complex robotic DP, including those that require SMV dissection and tunneling under the pancreatic neck, at the same time we gained lymph node dissection and reconstruction skills through robotic gastrectomies, before undertaking robotic PD. Finally, structured observation and multiple attending surgeon participation in each operation ensures shared progression along the learning curve.

General Techniques and Retraction

After placement of intravenous and intra-arterial lines, the patient is positioned and padded. Safe abdominal access through preferred technique is obtained; in our experience, Veress needle access at Palmer's point followed by optical trocar entry or placement of GelPOINT access platform through Pfannenstiel incision and use of

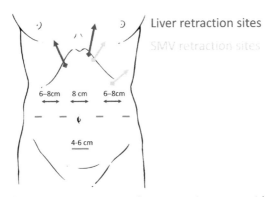

Liver retraction sites

SMV retraction sites

Fig. 1. Standardized robotic port placement for pancreatic surgery with external retractor placement for robotic PD.

the AirSeal System (CONMED, Largo, FL). Port placement is standardized (**Fig. 1**), with extraction performed through a small Pfannenstiel incision.

Consistent exposure of surgical field to identify and protect key anatomical structures is vital in MIP. We developed standardized external retraction techniques to facilitate adequate surgical exposure using a suture passer and clamping the retracted strings at the skin level.[15] Typical retraction placement is demonstrated in **Fig. 2**. A 10-cm Penrose drain is used for liver retraction with a 3-0 Vicryl suture in the center with the needle left in place, and 0-silk sutures at either end. The Vicryl at the midpoint of the drain is sutured to the diaphragmatic crus, and the silk sutures at either end are retracted externally at the xiphoid process, exposing the anterior stomach and porta hepatis. External retraction systems using the Nathanson or other devices have also been described. The stomach can be easily externally retracted with the placement of a Vicryl stitch on the posterior wall. For retraction of the SMV during this step of robotic PD, we place three vessel loops encircling the vessel and carefully externally retract this vessel to expose the lateral and posterior aspect of the SMA. This retraction technique can be viewed at: https://www.youtube.com/watch?v=48_bVFh2I3c

Distal Pancreatectomy

Current evidence and outcomes

As DP lacks the need for reconstruction, both laparoscopic and robotic DP have been widely adopted. MI DP is safe and feasible for benign and malignant indications.[20,23]

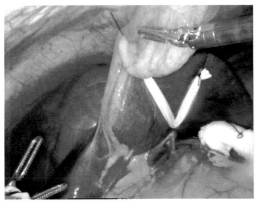

Fig. 2. Liver retractor (3–0 Vicryl suture in the middle, 0 silk sutures on either ends).

For PNETs in particular, retrospective matched cohort studies demonstrated similar disease-free survival after laparoscopic resection, with significantly decreased rates of postoperative complications and length of stay.[42] Retrospective analyses have consistently demonstrated laparoscopic DP is associated with lower blood loss and length of stay, improved postoperative quality of life, and similar costs, without appreciable increases in postoperative POPF, short-term complications, mortality, or rate of R0 resections in comparison with open approach.[17,43–46]

Randomized controlled data supports MI DP over the open approach. The LEOPARD-1 trial randomized one hundred and eight patients with left-sided pancreatic tumors, without evidence of vascular involvement, to MI DP (42 laparoscopic, 5 robotic) or open DP. Of note, patients were blinded to surgical approach using a large abdominal dressing. MI DP demonstrated decreased time to functional recovery (4 versus 6 days, $P < 0.001$), decreased rates of delayed gastric emptying (3 patients (6%) vs 11 patients (20%); $P = 0.04$) without a difference in rate of POPF (39% vs 23% for MIDP and open DP, respectively [$P = 0.07$]), or 90-day mortality. Follow-up analyses of cost and quality of life up to 1 year after surgery showed comparable costs after MI DP, with a probability of at least 0.654 of improved cost-effectiveness.[3,47] Of note, however, long-term follow-up (up to 3 years) after DP demonstrated no differences in overall quality of life between MI and open DP. The LAPOP trial is an unblinded, parallel group, single-center superiority trial between laparoscopic open DP.[48] Twenty-nine patients were randomized to each group, demonstrating improvements in length of stay (5 vs 6 days, $P = 0.007$) and blood loss (50 vs 100 mL, $P = 0.015$) for laparoscopic and open DP, respectively. No differences were observed between Clavien–-Dindo III + complications, rates of delayed gastric emptying or grade B/C POPF.[49]

In addition, retrospective studies have shown equivalent oncologic outcomes after MI DP compared with open although it is important to acknowledge that these retrospective studies may be subject to selection bias and that no randomized long-term survival data have been reported. The European Consortium on Minimally Invasive Pancreatic Surgery reported the results of a pan-European matched cohort study between MI and open DP in pancreatic ductal adenocarcinoma, matching 340 patients.[43] This study demonstrated decreases in median blood loss (200 vs 300 mL, $P = 0.001$) and length of stay (8 vs 9 days, $P < 0.001$), for MI versus open DP, respectively. No differences were seen in 90-day mortality (2% vs 3%) and Clavien–Dindo III + complications (18 vs 21%) for MI and open DP, respectively. Most importantly, no differences were observed in median overall survival between MI DP and open DP (28 vs 31 months, $P = 0.929$). However, MI DP was associated with higher rates of R0 resection (67% vs 58%, $P = 0.019$) and lower lymph node yield (14 vs 22, $P < 0.001$). As a result of these data, the same group is currently enrolling 258 patients in a multicenter, non-inferiority, randomized controlled trial between MI DP (laparoscopic or robotic) and open. Their primary outcome measure is the microscopically radical resection margin, and secondary outcomes include time to functional recovery and survival.[50] Several additional international trials are ongoing between MI and open DP, including a multicenter, non-inferiority, non-blinded randomized controlled trial in Korea, with primary endpoint of 2-year survival.[51] The DISPACT-2 trial in Germany is currently enrolling, randomizing 294 patients between MI and open DP, with a primary outcome measure of postoperative morbidity and mortality.[52]

Robotic versus laparoscopic DP has been examined in multiple recent meta-analyses. These studies reported lower rates of open conversion and shorter hospital stay, with higher rates of spleen preservation after robotic DP, and no differences between morbidity and POPF rate.[53–55] However, robotic DP was associated with higher operative time. In PNETs in particular, robotic DP is associated with improved splenic preservation compared with laparoscopic DP (65.3% vs 44.7%, $P < 0.0001$) in a retrospective analysis of 181 patients at four tertiary Italian referral centers.[56] This study also reported no differences in short- or long-term perioperative outcomes, including overall and disease-free survival. Cost favored the laparoscopic approach, with mean total costs of 9235 versus 11226 €, for the laparoscopic and robotic DP, respectively, $P < 0.0001$. Although these data likely represent selection bias, in appropriate hands both laparoscopic and robotic DP seem to be safe and effective options for the treatment of the spectrum of pancreatic tumors.

Technical approach to robotic distal pancreatectomy

Positioning and Abdominal Access: The patient is placed supine on the surgical bed, and all pressure points are padded. Surgical robot (daVinci Xi platform, Intuitive Surgical, USA) can be docked from either patient's side, with the arms rotated targeting cephalad. We begin by making the small Pfannenstiel incision to place the GelPort and AirSeal. Four additional robotic ports are placed at the midpoint level between anterior superior iliac spine and inferior costal margin, pneumoperitoneum is established at 10 to 15 mm Hg and should be maintained as low as feasible, and the patient is positioned at 10° to 15° in reverse Trendelenburg. Liposomal bupivacaine solution is used to perform a transversus abdominis plane block under laparoscopic direct vision.

Pancreatic Exposure: Liver retractor is placed first to allow dissection of the stomach. The lesser sac is entered below the gastroepiploic vessels, separating the stomach from the colon. This dissection is carried out using the Vessel Sealer all the way to the short gastric vessels toward the angle of His. Any posterior attachments of the stomach to the pancreas are then divided. The gastric retraction stitches are then placed to achieve excellent exposure of splenic hilum to complete separation of the spleen from the stomach. The splenic flexure is then mobilized from the inferior border of the pancreas, exposing the caudad portion of the spleen.

Tumor Identification: Minimally invasive ultrasound is then used to ensure proper identification of the pancreatic pathology.

Pancreatic Dissection: Inferior pancreatic dissection is first accomplished at the inferior pancreatic border along the retropancreatic fascial plane, widely established toward the splenic hilum, carefully avoiding injury to the insertion of the inferior mesenteric vein.[57] This plane continues cephalad to the layer of diaphragm to include splenic artery lymph nodes in the specimen. The dissection is carried medially depending on the relative location of the pathology. The pancreas, splenic vein, and artery are then elevated en bloc off the retroperitoneum. Umbilical tape is then passed through this tunnel to allow upward retraction of the specimen.

Splenic Vessel/Pancreatic Division: For tumors located at the tail or distal body of the pancreas, depending on the relative anatomic relationships of the splenic artery to the splenic vein/pancreas, these may be taken with one staple fire en bloc or separately. For tumors located at proximal body, pancreas tunneling above SMV/PV is required. We identify and follow the middle colic vein to identify the SMV to begin the pancreas tunneling. The common hepatic artery lymph node is dissected off to open the window to complete tunneling at cephalad. The pancreas is divided at the neck using a stapler (our preference is to use absorbable stapler reinforcement on blue load Echelon or SureForm stapler). The splenic artery is divided with clips/ties or a vascular load stapler, and the splenic vein is divided after secure ligation and clipping, or with a vascular load stapler. The remainder of the retroperitoneal attachments is divided in medial-to-lateral approach, and the specimen is removed via the Pfannenstiel incision in a protective bag.

Table 1 Post-pancreatectomy-enhanced recovery pathways		
	Pancreaticoduodenectomy	Distal Pancreatectomy
Regional anesthesia	+	+
Intraoperative fluids	Restrictive intra- and post-op	Restrictive intra- and post-op
NGT removal	POD 1	N/A
Foley catheter removal	POD 2	POD 1
Drain removal	POD 1 or 3 with DFA cutoffs (<661 U/L POD1, <141 U/L POD3)	POD 1 or 3(<661 U/L POD1, <141 U/L POD3)
Enoxaparin on discharge	+	+
Anticipated discharge	POD 4	POD 3

NGT, nasogastric tube; POD, postoperative day; DFA, drain fluid amlyase.
Adapted from Newton AD, Newhook TE, Bruno ML, et al. Iterative Changes in Risk-Stratified Pancreatectomy Clinical Pathways and Accelerated Discharge After Pancreaticoduodenectomy. J Gastrointest Surg 2022. https://doi.org/10.1007/s11605-021-05235-3.

Closure/Drainage/Recovery: A 19-French blake drain is placed through a right side port site near, but ideally not in contact with, the staple line. The omentum is to the left also the splenic bed carefully draped over the staple line to provide coverage and separation from the posterior stomach. The Pfannenstiel incision is closed. Postoperatively the patient is managed according to an enhanced recovery pathway (**Table 1**).[58]

Pancreaticoduodenectomy

Current evidence and outcomes
PD is technically demanding, with considerable challenges in dissection and reconstruction. Mortality from open PD has decreased over time, from near 25% in the 1960s and 1970s to less than 5% in recent years.[59] With both increased performance of PD and developments in minimally invasive surgery, interest in performance of MI PD has developed over the last 30 years. The first described laparoscopic PD was performed in 1994, and since that time performance MI PD has increased. Case-series and meta-analyses suggest that MI PD is associated with decreased blood loss, with similar mortality and complication rates.[60,61] In particular, Torphy and colleagues[62] reported data from the NCDB that suggests centers in the top fifth percentile for total PD volume, patients who underwent MI PD had decreased length of stay, with similar 30-day mortality, readmissions, margin status, and lymph node yield.

Three randomized controlled trials have evaluated laparoscopic versus open PD. In the PLOT trial, Palanivelu and colleagues randomized 64 patients to either laparoscopic or open PD, at one high-volume center in India. In this trial, although laparoscopic PD was associated with higher operative times, it was also associated with decreased length of stay (13 vs 7 days) and decreased blood loss (250 vs 401 mL), without differences in delayed gastric emptying, POPF, complications, or mortality.[4] In the PADULAP trial, Poves and colleagues randomized 66 patients to laparoscopic or open PD, demonstrating decreased length of stay (13.5 vs 17 days), decreased postoperative Clavien–Dindo III + complications (5 vs 11 patients), without differences in rates of margin positivity or lymph node yield. In the multicenter LEOPARD-2 trial, 105 patients were randomized to laparoscopic or open PD at four high-volume (20+) centers in the Netherlands. This trial was prematurely terminated due to prohibitively high 90-day mortality in the laparoscopic group (5/50 patients in the laparoscopic group vs 1/49 patients in the open group).[6]

No randomized controlled trial exists comparing robotic with laparoscopic PD. One would predict the theoretical advantages of robotic surgery, improved dexterity, three-dimensional visualization, and improved ergonomics and would translate into improved outcomes compared with laparoscopic PD. However, retrospective data suggest that robotic PD is a safe approach with acceptable perioperative outcomes. Nassour and colleagues[63] reported no differences between laparoscopic and robotic PD in the American College of Surgeons National Surgical Quality Improvement Program database. In addition, results from the National Cancer Database suggest no differences between laparoscopic and robotic PD in short-term outcomes (margin status, length of stay, and 90-day mortality) and long-term oncologic outcomes (median overall survival, 1- and 3- year survival).[64] In a multi-institutional analysis comparing robotic and open PD among surgeons beyond the learning curve, Zureikat and colleagues[65] reported reductions in blood loss (median difference -181 mL, $P = 0.04$) and major complications (adjusted odds $= 0.64$, $P = 0.003$) after robotic surgery at the cost of higher operative time (median difference $+75.4$ minutes, $P = 0.01$), with no relevant differences in POPF, wound infection, length of stay, or readmission.

Prospective evidence supporting the long-term oncologic quality of robotic PD is lacking, though smaller retrospective studies suggest equivalence. In another National Cancer Database, robotic PD was associated with improved lymph node yield (OR 3.055, $P < 0.0001$) and increased rates of receipt of adjuvant therapy (OR 2.454, $P < 0.001$) after administration of neoadjuvant chemotherapy in pancreatic adenocarcinoma.[66] The PORTAL trial is currently enrolling, randomizing 244 patients with to open versus robotic PD in high-volume centers in China.[67] Primary outcome measures of this study will be time to functional recovery, and percentage of patients who receive adjuvant chemotherapy at 8 weeks in the pancreatic adenocarcinoma sub-cohort. This and other prospective trials are needed to determine the safety and oncologic outcomes of robotic PD compared with open.

Technical approach to robotic pancreaticoduodenectomy

Patient Positioning/Pancreatic Exposure: Patient positioning, pancreatic exposure, and gastric/hepatic retraction are performed in the same fashion as in the robotic DP. In addition, gallbladder is sutured to abdominal wall to facilitate posterior portal exposure.

Lesser Sac Dissection and Kocherization: After division of the omentum to enter the lesser sac, we continue dissection along the mesocolon layer toward patient's right. Then, we identify and follow middle colic vein toward the superior mesenteric vein and gastrocolic trunk. Accessory colic veins are divided with hemo-lock clips and/ or the Vessel Sealer. SMV dissection is continued cephalad under the head of the pancreas. The right colon is completely mobilized down to the cecum to facilitate posterior SMV exposure, and then an extended Kocher maneuver with the mobilization of the duodenum and pancreatic head off the IVC is performed to expose left renal vein and the root of SMA. Any suspicious or enlarged aortocaval lymph nodes are sampled for immediate assessment as needed.

Antrectomy: The omentum is then dissected off the stomach, and the gastroepiploic arcade is divided at the point of gastric transection. We then divide the stomach with staplers.

Portal Dissection: We perform a complete hepatic arterial lymph node dissection (#8a/#8p), identifying the gastroduodenal artery and clipping it three times, and confirming hepatic artery flow is intact. We then define medial border of hepatic artery

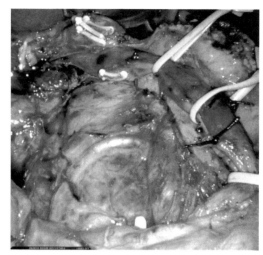

Fig. 3. External SMV retraction facilitating periadventitial SMA dissection.

lymph node dissection, with intent to be connected with future SMA dissection posteriorly. We continue posterior hepatic artery dissection and portal vein dissection. We reflect all periportal (#12) lymph nodes down with the specimen.

Ligament of Treitz Mobilization: We then flip the transverse colon and divide the jejunum using stapler approximately 15 to 20 cm distal to the ligament of Treitz, where we can have enough length of mesentery to allow tension-free anastomoses. We divide the small bowel mesentery with the vessel sealer and flip the duodenum to the right side of the specimen.

Pancreatic transection and retroperitoneal dissection: Using upward tension, we carefully develop the portal vein/SMV tunnel, retracting the pancreas superiorly with passed umbilical tape. We then divide the pancreas using bipolar energy. Once the pancreas is divided, we place vessel loops around the SMV for external tension to obtain adequate SMA exposure (**Fig. 3**). All small branches are divided off the SMV/portal vein, except the posterior superior pancreatoduodenal vein ("the vein of Belcher") which should be preserved until all arterial supply to the head of the pancreas is divided to avoid specimen congestion. Periadventitial SMA dissection is then performed caudad to cephalad, identifying and dividing all inferior pancreaticoduodenal branches with clips and devices. Finally, all retroperitoneal attachments of the specimen are divided, and the posterior hepatic artery lymph node is swept upward with the specimen. Gallbladder is taken down in top-down fashion to the root of cystic duct. The bile duct is divided to free the specimen en bloc. Specimen is extracted in plastic bag. Pancreatic and bile duct margins are routinely sent to immediate pathologic assessment.

The small bowl limb is pulled through the avascular window of mesocolon, right to the middle colic artery, for reconstruction.

Hepaticojejunostomy: Techniques being used for HJ reconstruction varies, depending on the size of the duct. For ducts with large caliber, running sutures using 4-0 stratafix with RB-1 needle is appropriate and time saving. For small ducts (<3 mm), interrupted sutures using 5-0 PDS are recommended at least for anterior row to avoid inadvertent back-wall stich and anastomotic stenosis.

Pancreatico-jejunostomy: We use modified Blumgart techniques for PJ anasto-mosis. We place trans-pancreatic prolene U-stitches through the pancreas after first going through the bowel with pledgets. For small size duct (<3 mm), we use a small (18–22 Fr) angiocatheter to dilate the pancreatic duct. Then, we sew the back row with three interrupted 5-0 PDS suture, with the knots inside the duct. Three stitches are placed anteriorly, with the knots on the outside of the duct. Using the previously placed prolene U-stitches, the bowel is folded over the top to create our outer row. These are secured down with pledgets using Lapra-Ty device (Ethicon, New Jersey) under appropriate tension.[68]

Gastrojejunostomy: We perform an antecolic stapled gastrojejunostomy approxi-mately 30 to 40 cm downstream of the hepaticojejunostomy first making a gastrotomy and enterotomy, and using a 60 mm stapling device to create a common channel. The common enterotomy is oversewn with running 3-0 V-lock suture.

Drain placement: Two 19-French round Blake drains are placed through the abdom-inal wall: one from the patient's right just over Morrison's pouch behind the pancreatic and biliary anastomoses and one anterior to the pancreas from the left side.

Pancreatic Enucleation

Pancreatic enucleation, particularly for low-risk endocrine lesions of the pancreas such as small insulinomas, has gained traction as a parenchymal sparing approach. Although enucleation may broadly be associated with increased rate of POPF, when applied in high-volume center this increased risk seems to be abrogated.[69] Mini-mally invasive enucleation, including laparoscopic and robotic approaches, has been described in retrospective series. In particular, for PNETs, several retrospective series of minimally invasive enucleation have been published supporting this technique. Ben-edetto and colleagues[70] described a series of 12 patients who underwent robotic enucleation, with 1/12 developing clinically relevant POPF, and no recurrence at a me-dian follow-up of 17 months. In a large multicenter matched cohort analysis, Tian and colleagues[71] compared 187 open PNET enucleations with 61 performed robotically. There were no observed differences in POPF (17.0% open vs 10% robotic) or rates of grade III + Clavien–Dindo complications (3% robotic vs 10% open) and decreased blood loss in the robotic group (80 mL vs. 32.5 mL, open and robotic, respectively).

General criteria for pancreatic enucleation include benign imaging appearance, size less than 2 cm and adequate distance from the pancreatic duct to prevent injury.[72] Careful planning and patient counseling is needed before performance of pancreatic enucleation, with counseling regarding the need to convert to a formal pancreatic resection based on intraoperative characteristics.

SUMMARY

Minimally invasive techniques in pancreatectomy are increasingly being used. Mini-mally invasive DP seems to be the standard approach for most low-grade distal pancreatic lesions, and ongoing trials may further bolster its use in pancreatic adeno-carcinoma. However, minimally invasive PD remains controversial, with selected high-volume centers reporting successful case series. Maintaining high levels of oncologic excellence, with negative-margin resection remains the challenge facing wide adop-tion of minimally invasive PD. Adherence to the key technical standards of pancreatic resection during a minimally invasive approach, while simultaneously traversing the learning curve of these procedures is the key to their ultimate success. Ongoing hos-pital- and national-level planning should play a role in the development of safe MIP programs.

CONFLICTS OF INTEREST

None to declare.

REFERENCES

1. Hoehn RS, Nassour I, Adam MA, et al. National Trends in Robotic Pancreas Surgery. J Gastrointest Surg 2021;25(4):983–90.
2. Stewart CL, Ituarte PHG, Melstrom KA, et al. Robotic surgery trends in general surgical oncology from the National Inpatient Sample. Surg Endosc 2019;33(8): 2591–601.
3. de Rooij T, van Hilst J, van Santvoort H, et al. Minimally invasive versus open distal pancreatectomy (LEOPARD): a multicenter patient-blinded randomized controlled trial. Ann Surg 2019;269(1):2–9.
4. Palanivelu C, Senthilnathan P, Sabnis SC, et al. Randomized clinical trial of laparoscopic versus open pancreatoduodenectomy for periampullary tumours. Br J Surg 2017;104(11):1443–50.
5. Poves I, Burdío F, Morató O, et al. Comparison of perioperative outcomes between laparoscopic and open approach for pancreatoduodenectomy: the padulap randomized controlled trial. Ann Surg 2018;268(5):731–9.
6. van Hilst J, de Rooij T, Bosscha K, et al. Laparoscopic versus open pancreatoduodenectomy for pancreatic or periampullary tumours (LEOPARD-2): a multicentre, patient-blinded, randomised controlled phase 2/3 trial. Lancet Gastroenterol Hepatol 2019;4(3):199–207.
7. Kim J, Hwang HK, Lee WJ, et al. Minimally invasive vs open pancreatectomy for nonfunctioning pancreatic neuroendocrine tumors. World J Gastrointest Oncol 2020;12(10):1133–45.
8. Zhang X-F, Lopez-Aguiar AG, Poultsides G, et al. Minimally invasive versus open distal pancreatectomy for pancreatic neuroendocrine tumors: an analysis from the U.S. neuroendocrine tumor study group. J Surg Oncol 2019;120(2):231–40.
9. Ferraro V, Tedeschi M, Laera L, et al. The role of laparoscopic surgery in localized pancreatic neuroendocrine tumours. Curr Treat Options Oncol 2021;22(4):27.
10. de Rooij T, van Hilst J, Topal B, et al. Outcomes of a multicenter training program in laparoscopic pancreatoduodenectomy (LAELAPS-2). Ann Surg 2019;269(2): 344–50.
11. de Rooij T, van Hilst J, Boerma D, et al. Impact of a nationwide training program in minimally invasive distal pancreatectomy (LAELAPS). Ann Surg 2016;264(5): 754–62.
12. Zwart MJW, Nota CLM, de Rooij T, et al. Outcomes of a multicenter training program in robotic pancreatoduodenectomy (LAELAPS-3). Ann Surg 2022. https://doi.org/10.1097/SLA.0000000000004783.
13. Stocchi L, Nelson H, Sargent DJ, et al. Impact of surgical and pathologic variables in rectal cancer: a United States community and cooperative group report. J Clin Oncol 2001;19(18):3895–902.
14. Katz MHG, Merchant NB, Brower S, et al. Standardization of surgical and pathologic variables is needed in multicenter trials of adjuvant therapy for pancreatic cancer: results from the ACOSOG Z5031 trial. Ann Surg Oncol 2011;18(2): 337–44.
15. Ikoma N, Kim MP, Tzeng C-WD, et al. External retraction technique for robotic pancreatoduodenectomy. J Am Coll Surg 2020;231(5):e8–10.
16. U.S. Food & Drug Administration website, Caution when using robotically-assisted surgical devices in women's health including mastectomy and other cancer-

related surgeries: FDA safety communication. Access URL: https://www.fda.gov/medical-devices/safety-communications/update-caution-robotically-assisted-surgical-devices-mastectomy-fda-safety-communication, 2021, FDA.

17. Braga M, Pecorelli N, Ferrari D, et al. Results of 100 consecutive laparoscopic distal pancreatectomies: postoperative outcome, cost-benefit analysis, and quality of life assessment. Surg Endosc 2015;29(7):1871–8.

18. Zureikat AH, Beane JD, Zenati MS, et al. 500 Minimally invasive robotic pancreatoduodenectomies: one decade of optimizing performance. Ann Surg 2021;273(5):966–72.

19. Song KB, Kim SC, Park JB, et al. Single-center experience of laparoscopic left pancreatic resection in 359 consecutive patients: changing the surgical paradigm of left pancreatic resection. Surg Endosc 2011;25(10):3364–72.

20. Asbun HJ, Moekotte AL, Vissers FL, et al. The miami international evidence-based guidelines on minimally invasive pancreas resection. Ann Surg 2020;271(1):1–14.

21. Gianotti L, Besselink MG, Sandini M, et al. Nutritional support and therapy in pancreatic surgery: a position paper of the International Study Group on Pancreatic Surgery (ISGPS). Surgery 2018;164(5):1035–48.

22. Lambert JE, Hayes LD, Keegan TJ, et al. The impact of prehabilitation on patient outcomes in hepatobiliary, colorectal, and upper gastrointestinal cancer surgery: a PRISMA-accordant meta-analysis. Ann Surg 2021;274(1):70–7.

23. de Rooij T, Besselink MG, Shamali A, et al. Pan-European survey on the implementation of minimally invasive pancreatic surgery with emphasis on cancer. HPB 2016;18(2):170–6.

24. Jayaraman S, Gonen M, Brennan MF, et al. Laparoscopic distal pancreatectomy: evolution of a technique at a single institution. J Am Coll Surgeons 2010;211(4):503–9.

25. Klompmaker S, Zoggel D van, Watkins AA, et al. Nationwide evaluation of patient selection for minimally invasive distal pancreatectomy using american college of surgeons' national quality improvement program. Ann Surg 2017;266(6):1055–61.

26. Scheib SA, Tanner E, Green IC, et al. Laparoscopy in the morbidly obese: physiologic considerations and surgical techniques to optimize success. J Minimally Invasive Gynecol 2014;21(2):182–95.

27. van Wissen J, Bakker N, Doodeman HJ, et al. Preoperative methods to reduce liver volume in bariatric surgery: a systematic review. Obes Surg 2016;26(2):251–6.

28. Kim JH, Gonzalez-Heredia R, Daskalaki D, et al. Totally replaced right hepatic artery in pancreaticoduodenectomy: is this anatomical condition a contraindication to minimally invasive surgery? HPB 2016;18(7):580–5.

29. Alsfasser G, Leicht H, Günster C, et al. Volume-outcome relationship in pancreatic surgery. Br J Surg 2016;103(1):136–43.

30. Birkmeyer JD, Siewers AE, Finlayson EVA, et al. Hospital volume and surgical mortality in the United States. N Engl J Med 2002;346(15):1128–37.

31. Busweiler LAD, Dikken JL, Henneman D, et al. The influence of a composite hospital volume on outcomes for gastric cancer surgery: a Dutch population-based study. J Surg Oncol 2017;115(6):738–45.

32. Wang M, Meng L, Cai Y, et al. Learning curve for laparoscopic pancreaticoduodenectomy: a CUSUM analysis. J Gastrointest Surg 2016;20(5):924–35.

33. Kim S, Yoon Y-S, Han H-S, et al. Evaluation of a single surgeon's learning curve of laparoscopic pancreaticoduodenectomy: risk-adjusted cumulative summation analysis. Surg Endosc 2021;35(6):2870–8.
34. Haney CM, Karadza E, Limen EF, et al. Training and learning curves in minimally invasive pancreatic surgery: from simulation to mastery. J Pancreatology 2020; 3(2):101–10.
35. Boone BA, Zenati M, Hogg ME, et al. Assessment of quality outcomes for robotic pancreaticoduodenectomy: identification of the learning curve. JAMA Surg 2015; 150(5):416–22.
36. Mark Knab L, Zenati MS, Khodakov A, et al. Evolution of a novel robotic training curriculum in a complex general surgical oncology fellowship. Ann Surg Oncol 2018;25(12):3445–52.
37. Hogg ME, Tam V, Zenati M, et al. Mastery-based virtual reality robotic simulation curriculum: the first step toward operative robotic proficiency. J Surg Educ 2017; 74(3):477–85.
38. Tam V, Zenati M, Novak S, et al. Robotic pancreatoduodenectomy biotissue curriculum has validity and improves technical performance for surgical oncology fellows. J Surg Educ 2017;74(6):1057–65.
39. Harris BR, Musgrove KA, Hogg ME, et al. Formal robotic training reduces the learning curve of robotic pancreaticoduodenectomy. HPB 2020;22:S132.
40. Chan KS, Wang ZK, Syn N, et al. Learning curve of laparoscopic and robotic pancreas resections: a systematic review. Surgery 2021;170(1):194–206.
41. Shakir M, Boone BA, Polanco PM, et al. The learning curve for robotic distal pancreatectomy: an analysis of outcomes of the first 100 consecutive cases at a high-volume pancreatic centre. HPB (Oxford) 2015;17(7):580–6.
42. Partelli S, Andreasi V, Rancoita PMV, et al. Outcomes after distal pancreatectomy for neuroendocrine neoplasms: a retrospective comparison between minimally invasive and open approach using propensity score weighting. Surg Endosc 2021;35(1):165–73.
43. van Hilst J, de Rooij T, Klompmaker S, et al. Minimally Invasive versus Open Distal Pancreatectomy for Ductal Adenocarcinoma (DIPLOMA): A Pan-European Propensity Score Matched Study. Ann Surg 2019;269(1):10–7.
44. Tran Cao HS, Lopez N, Chang DC, et al. Improved Perioperative Outcomes With Minimally Invasive Distal Pancreatectomy: Results From a Population-Based Analysis. JAMA Surg 2014;149(3):237–43.
45. Riviere D, Gurusamy KS, Kooby DA, et al. Laparoscopic versus open distal pancreatectomy for pancreatic cancer. Cochrane Database Syst Rev 2016;4: CD011391.
46. Yang D-J, Xiong J-J, Lu H-M, et al. The oncological safety in minimally invasive versus open distal pancreatectomy for pancreatic ductal adenocarcinoma: a systematic review and meta-analysis. Sci Rep 2019;9(1):1159.
47. Korrel M, Roelofs A, van Hilst J, et al. Long-Term Quality of Life after Minimally Invasive vs Open Distal Pancreatectomy in the LEOPARD Randomized Trial. J Am Coll Surg 2021;233(6):730–9.e9.
48. Björnsson B, Sandström P, Larsson AL, et al. Laparoscopic versus open distal pancreatectomy (LAPOP): study protocol for a single center, nonblinded, randomized controlled trial. Trials 2019;20:356.
49. Björnsson B, Larsson AL, Hjalmarsson C, et al. Comparison of the duration of hospital stay after laparoscopic or open distal pancreatectomy: randomized controlled trial. Br J Surg 2020;107(10):1281–8.

50. van Hilst J, Korrel M, Lof S, et al. Minimally invasive versus open distal pancreatectomy for pancreatic ductal adenocarcinoma (DIPLOMA): study protocol for a randomized controlled trial. Trials 2021;22(1):608.
51. Multicenter Prospective Randomized Controlled Clinical Trial for Comparison Between Laparoscopic and Open Distal Pancreatectomy for Ductal Adenocarcinoma of the Pancreatic Body and Tail. clinicaltrials.gov; 2019. Access URL: https://clinicaltrials.gov/ct2/sho the Pancreatic Body and Tail. clinicaltrials.gov; 2019. Access URL: https://clinicaltrials.gov/ct2/show/NCT03957135.
52. Probst P, Schuh F, Dörr-Harim C, et al. Protocol for a randomised controlled trial to compare postoperative complications between minimally invasive and open DIStal PAnCreaTectomy (DISPACT-2 trial). BMJ Open 2021;11(2):e047867.
53. Kamarajah SK, Sutandi N, Robinson SR, et al. Robotic versus conventional laparoscopic distal pancreatic resection: a systematic review and meta-analysis. HPB (Oxford) 2019;21(9):1107–18.
54. Guerrini GP, Lauretta A, Belluco C, et al. Robotic versus laparoscopic distal pancreatectomy: an up-to-date meta-analysis. BMC Surg 2017;17(1):105.
55. Hong S, Song KB, Madkhali AA, et al. Robotic versus laparoscopic distal pancreatectomy for left-sided pancreatic tumors: a single surgeon's experience of 228 consecutive cases. Surg Endosc 2020;34(6):2465–73.
56. Alfieri S, Butturini G, Boggi U, et al. Short-term and long-term outcomes after robot-assisted versus laparoscopic distal pancreatectomy for pancreatic neuroendocrine tumors (pNETs): a multicenter comparative study. Langenbecks Arch Surg 2019;404(4):459–68.
57. Yang JD, Ishikawa K, Hwang HP, et al. Retropancreatic fascia is absent along the pancreas facing the superior mesenteric artery: a histological study using elderly donated cadavers. Surg Radiol Anat 2013;35(5):403–10.
58. Newton AD, Newhook TE, Bruno ML, et al. Iterative Changes in Risk-Stratified Pancreatectomy Clinical Pathways and Accelerated Discharge After Pancreaticoduodenectomy. J Gastrointest Surg 2022. https://doi.org/10.1007/s11605-021-05235-3.
59. Cameron JL, Riall TS, Coleman J, et al. One thousand consecutive pancreaticoduodenectomies. Ann Surg 2006;244(1):10–5.
60. Chen K, Pan Y, Liu X-L, et al. Minimally invasive pancreaticoduodenectomy for periampullary disease: a comprehensive review of literature and meta-analysis of outcomes compared with open surgery. BMC Gastroenterol 2017;17(1):120.
61. Wang S, Shi N, You L, et al. Minimally invasive surgical approach versus open procedure for pancreaticoduodenectomy: a systematic review and meta-analysis. Medicine (Baltimore) 2017;96(50):e8619.
62. Torphy RJ, Friedman C, Halpern A, et al. Comparing short-term and oncologic outcomes of minimally invasive versus open pancreaticoduodenectomy across low and high volume centers. Ann Surg 2019;270(6):1147–55.
63. Nassour I, Wang SC, Porembka MR, et al. Robotic versus laparoscopic pancreaticoduodenectomy: a NSQIP analysis. J Gastrointest Surg 2017;21(11):1784–92.
64. Nassour I, Choti MA, Porembka MR, et al. Robotic-assisted versus laparoscopic pancreaticoduodenectomy: oncological outcomes. Surg Endosc 2018;32(6):2907–13.
65. Zureikat AH, Postlewait LM, Liu Y, et al. a multi-institutional comparison of perioperative outcomes of robotic and open pancreaticoduodenectomy. Ann Surg 2016;264(4):640–9.

66. Nassour I, Tohme S, Hoehn R, et al. Safety and oncologic efficacy of robotic compared to open pancreaticoduodenectomy after neoadjuvant chemotherapy for pancreatic cancer. Surg Endosc 2021;35(5):2248–54.

67. Robotic versus Open Pancreatoduodenectomy for Pancreatic and Periampullary Tumors (PORTAL): a study protocol for a multicenter phase III non-inferiority randomized controlled trial | Trials | Full Text. Available at: https://trialsjournal. biomedcentral.com/articles/10.1186/s13063-021-05939-6/figures/1. Accessed January 22, 2022.

68. Nagakawa Y, Takishita C, Hijikata Y, et al. Blumgart method using LAPRA-TY clips facilitates pancreaticojejunostomy in laparoscopic pancreaticoduodenectomy. Medicine (Baltimore) 2020;99(10):e19474.

69. Hüttner FJ, Koessler-Ebs J, Hackert T, et al. Meta-analysis of surgical outcome after enucleation versus standard resection for pancreatic neoplasms. Br J Surg 2015;102(9):1026–36.

70. Di Benedetto F, Magistri P, Ballarin R, et al. Ultrasound-guided robotic enucleation of pancreatic neuroendocrine tumors. Surg Innov 2019;26(1):37–45.

71. Tian F, Hong X-F, Wu W-M, et al. Propensity score-matched analysis of robotic versus open surgical enucleation for small pancreatic neuroendocrine tumours. Br J Surg 2016;103(10):1358–64.

72. Pitt SC, Pitt HA, Baker MS, et al. Small pancreatic and periampullary neuroendocrine tumors: resect or enucleate? J Gastrointest Surg 2009;13(9):1692–8.

Status of Surveillance and Nonsurgical Therapy for Small Nonfunctioning Pancreatic Neuroendocrine Tumors

Dirk-Jan van Beek, MD, PhD, MSc[a], Anna Vera D. Verschuur, MD[b],
Lodewijk A.A. Brosens, MD, PhD[c], Gerlof D. Valk, MD, PhD[d],
Carolina R.C. Pieterman, MD, PhD[d],*,[1], Menno R. Vriens, MD, PhD[a],[1]

KEYWORDS

- Pancreatic neuroendocrine tumors • Active surveillance
- Multiple endocrine neoplasia type 1 • Prognostic factors • EUS-Guided intervention

Continued

INTRODUCTION

Pancreatic neuroendocrine tumors (PNETs) are rare tumors with an estimated incidence of less than 1 per 100,000 people in Western countries.[1] Owing to increasing use and sensitivity of contemporary imaging studies, their incidence is rising. Surgical resection is the only curative treatment; however, complication rates are high. Small nonfunctioning (NF)-PNETs generally have an indolent natural course and prognosis is good even without upfront surgical resection. However, in a subset of these small tumors, metastases do occur. To be able to truly personalize treatment of NF-PNETs, novel prognostic factors are needed that will enable identification of those patients or tumors with high risk of metastases allowing early and aggressive targeted intervention. At the same time, low-risk tumors could be followed with active surveillance with a risk-dependent frequency. Nonsurgical treatment options that would allow early treatment of PNETs without the complications associated with surgery could lead to an important paradigm shift in the management of these tumors. This review provides an up-to-date overview of the status of surveillance and nonsurgical

[a] Department of Endocrine Surgical Oncology, University Medical Center Utrecht, Internal Mail Number G.04.228, PO Box 85500, Utrecht 3508 GA, the Netherlands; [b] Department of Pathology, University Medical Center Utrecht, Internal Mail Number G02.5.26, PO Box 85500, Utrecht 3508 GA, the Netherlands; [c] Department of Pathology, University Medical Center Utrecht, Internal Mail Number G4.02.06, PO Box 85500, Utrecht 3508 GA, the Netherlands; [d] Department of Endocrine Oncology, University Medical Center Utrecht, Internal Mail Number Q.05.4.300, PO Box 85500, Utrecht 3508 GA, the Netherlands
[1] These authors share senior authorship.
* Corresponding author.
E-mail address: c.r.c.pieterman@umcutrecht.nl
Twitter: @annaveraverschu (A.V.D.V.); @pieterman_carla (C.R.C.P.)

Surg Oncol Clin N Am 32 (2023) 343–371
https://doi.org/10.1016/j.soc.2022.10.010
surgonc.theclinics.com

Continued

KEY POINTS

- In both sporadic and Multiple Endocrine Neoplasia type 1 (MEN1)-related nonfunctional pancreatic neuroendocrine tumors (NF-PNETs), the most important and clinically actionable prognostic factors to guide management are tumor size, tumor growth, and tumor grade (World Health Organization).
- Surgical resection is recommended for sporadic and MEN1-related NF-PNET >2 cm in surgically fit patients.
- For patients with sporadic, asymptomatic G1 NF-PNETs <2 cm, initial active surveillance is a safe alternative to surgical resection on a group level. Identifying the individual patient with a small NF-PNET that potentially benefits from early surgical resection remains challenging. For patients with MEN1, an active surveillance strategy is usually followed until NF-PNETs reach 2 cm in size. Grade 2 tumors provide an indication for upfront surgery in smaller tumors.
- There is an urgent need for novel prognostic factors for small sporadic and MEN1-related NF-PNETs that will enable personalized decision-making for active surveillance or upfront surgery and guide decisions to intervene during active surveillance. Alpha-thalassemia/mental retardation X-linked/death domain-associated protein 6 and alternative lengthening of telomeres are promising novel tissue-based markers in this regard.
- At present, nonsurgical treatment options for small NF-PNETs are not considered an alternative to surgery. They are mainly used for those patients unfit for surgery or unwilling to undergo surgery.

interventions for both sporadic and multiple endocrine neoplasia type 1 (MEN1)-related small (<2 cm) nonmetastasized NF-PNETs.

BACKGROUND

PNETs represent less than 5% of all pancreatic tumors. Most of the PNETs (>80%) are not associated with hormonal syndromes and are referred to as NF-PNETs.[2] Data from the Surveillance, Epidemiology, and End Results database, show that the median overall survival of localized, regional and distant disease was approximately 230, 90 and 20 months, respectively.[1] Management of NF-PNETs is aimed at preventing metastases.

Most of the PNETs occur sporadically, whereas approximately 5% to 10% occur as part of a hereditary syndrome. MEN1, with an estimated prevalence of 1 in 20,000 to 1 in 40,000, is the most important hereditary syndrome associated with PNETs.[3] MEN1 is autosomal dominant and is caused by germline mutations in the tumor suppressor gene *MEN1* located on chromosome 11q13.[4] For an overview of the manifestations of MEN1 (**Fig. 1, Table 1**). Three out of four patients with MEN1 will have been diagnosed with a PNET by the age of 80, and malignant PNETs are the most important cause of disease-related mortality in MEN1.[5–7] MEN1-related PNETs are almost always multifocal and most are NF. Patients with MEN1 are advised to undergo screening to detect NF-PNETs at an early stage.[8] The goals of screening are to allow timely intervention to prevent the occurrence of metastases while preserving as much pancreatic tissue as possible and maintaining a good quality-of-life.

The North American Neuroendocrine Tumor Society (NANETS), European Neuroendocrine Tumor Society (ENETS), and the National Comprehensive Cancer Network (NCCN), provide guidelines or consensus statements on the management of PNETs, both sporadic and MEN1-related.[2,9–11] In addition, there are MEN1 specific guidelines

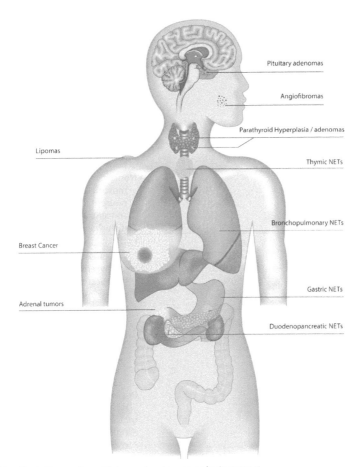

Fig. 1. Manifestations of multiple endocrine neoplasia type 1.

and consensus statements.[8,12] **Table 2** summarizes their main recommendations. The clinical practice guidelines for MEN1 (2012) are currently being revised.[8]

Sporadic Nonfunctional Pancreatic Neuroendocrine Tumors

Diagnostic workup

Owing to limited diagnostic accuracy, the NANETS guidelines do not recommend the use of nonspecific biochemical markers such as chromogranin A (CgA) and pancreastatin for the diagnosis of NF-PNETs.[2] Hence, imaging plays a pivotal role in the diagnosis, localization and staging of NF-PNETs. Anatomic imaging studies such as computed tomography (CT) or MRI are recommended for evaluation. If there is doubt about the PNET diagnosis, endoscopic ultrasound (EUS) with fine-needle aspiration (FNA) can be performed. Somatostatin-receptor positron emission tomography (SSTR-PET) with 68Ga-labeled DOTA-peptide somatostatin analogs is the best imaging modality for the detection of metastatic disease in patients with NF-PNETs and outperforms [11]In-pentreotide scintigraphy.[9,13] Combined with CT or MRI, it provides both essential anatomic and functional information. The workup of all patients with sporadic NF-PNETs should include anatomic imaging (CT or MRI) and 68Ga-labeled SSTR-PET (**Fig. 2**).[14]

Table 1
Manifestations of multiple endocrine neoplasia type 1

	Estimated Penetrance	Signs and Symptoms
PRIMARY HYPERPARATHYROIDISM	>95%	In patients prospectively screened often asymptomatic. Classic symptoms: Polyuria, polydipsia, gastro-intestinal complaints (eg, nausea, constipation, abdominal pain), pancreatitis, urolithiasis, decreased bone mineral density. Nonspecific symptoms: fatigue, musculoskeletal complaints, neuropsychiatric symptoms, concentration and sleep disturbances.
DUODENOPANCREATIC NEUROENDOCRINE TUMORS Nonfunctioning Insulinoma Gastrinoma Other rare functioning tumors	>80% >80% 10% to 15% 30% <5%	Usually asymptomatic, large tumors can cause symptoms by mass effect. Hypoglycemia: adrenergic symptoms (tachycardia, jitteriness, sweating, pale skin), and neuroglycopenic symptoms (altered mental status, irritability). Symptoms relieved by glucose intake. GERD, (PPI-responsive) diarrhea, abdominal pain, nausea/vomiting, weight loss, peptic ulcer disease, ZES. Depending on the hormone production. for example, extreme watery diarrhea (VIP); diabetes, steatorrhea and cholelithiasis (somatostatin); necrolytic migratory erythema, diabetes, weight loss (glucagon)
PITUITARY ADENOMAS Nonfunctioning Prolactinoma Other functioning PAs	50% 36% to 48% 30% to 80% <10%	Often asymptomatic micro-adenomas. Macro-adenomas may cause complaints by local mass effect such as visual field defects, headache, cranial nerve palsy and hypopituitarism. Females: galactorrhea, hypogonadism leading to amenorrhea and infertility Males: hypogonadism leading to impotence, lack of libido, infertility; rarely galactorrhea Depending hormone: acromegaly/ gigantism (GH), Cushing syndrome (ACTH), hypogonadism/ovarian hyperstimulation (FSH/LH), hyperthyroidism (TSH)
Neuroendocrine tumors of the lung	25%	Usually asymptomatic. Dyspnea, cough, hemoptysis, pneumonia may occur.

(continued on next page)

Table 1
(continued)

	Estimated Penetrance	Signs and Symptoms
Neuroendocrine tumors of the thymus	<10%	Symptoms of local mass effect in advanced stages. Rarely ectopic hormone production, then mostly ectopic ACTH leading to Cushing syndrome.
Neuroendocrine tumors of the stomach	<10%	Only seen in patients with ZES. Usually small and asymptomatic.
Adrenal adenomas Nonfunctioning Functioning	20% to 70%	Most adenomas are nonfunctioning and asymptomatic. Cortisol-producing adenomas may lead to Cushing syndrome, primary hyperaldosteronism can lead to therapy-resistant hypertension.
Breast cancer	Tbd	Palpable lump.
Skin lesions Collagenomas Angiofibromas	60% to 80%	May cause local symptoms.

Capitalized manifestations are the cardinal manifestations of MEN1, also known as "the three Ps".

Abbreviations: ACTH, adrenocorticotrophic hormone; FSH/LH, follicle stimulating hormone/luteinizing hormone; GERD, gastro-esophageal reflux disease; GH, growth hormone; PA, pituitary adenoma; PPI, proton-pump inhibitors tbd to be determined; TSH, thyroid stimulating hormone; VIP, vasoactive intestinal peptide, ZES, zollinger-ellison syndrome.

Data from Thakker et al., Clinical Practice guidelines for MEN1, JCEM 2012[8]; Pieterman et al., Update on the clinical management of multiple endocrine neoplasia type 1, Clin Endocrinol 2022[79]; Pieterman et al., MEN1, Endotext 2022.[80]

Surgical indications

Indications for surgery are primarily guided by size; all guidelines recommend surgical resection of NF-PNETs of 2 cm or larger.[9–11] For tumors <2 cm surgical indications vary between guidelines.

The ENETS guideline recommends operative resections for NF-PNETs <2 cm in case of World Health Organization (WHO) grade (G)2, symptoms, or patient preferences.[10] The NANETS consensus statement suggests individualized care for NF-PNET 1 to 2 cm taking age, comorbidities, tumor growth, the estimated risk of symptom development, tumor grade, the extent of surgical resection required, the patient's wishes, and access to long-term follow-up into account.[9] The NCCN guidelines suggest resection for invasive or node-positive PNETs <2 cm and states that the final decision should be based on estimated surgical risk, site of tumor, and patient comorbidities.[11]

Active surveillance for nonfunctional pancreatic neuroendocrine tumors <2 cm

Guidelines leave room for an individualized and nonsurgical management for NF-PNETs <2 cm (see **Table 2**). For these tumors, controversy exists regarding the benefit of surgery over active surveillance considering the high and procedure-dependent risk of complications.[15]

No randomized controlled trials have compared surgical resection with active surveillance to date. Multiple retrospective cohort studies have investigated active surveillance for NF-PNETs, of which some were included in two systematic reviews assessing active surveillance for NF-PNETs (**Table 3**).[16,17] They conclude that active

Table 2
Guideline recommendations for the management of sporadic and multiple endocrine neoplasia type 1–related nonfunctional pancreatic neuroendocrine tumor

Sporadic NF-PNET	Localization and Staging	Biopsy	Indication for Surgery	Surveillance
ENETS 2016	CT/MRI EUS ^{68}Ga-labeled somatostatin analogues with PET/CT	EUS-guided biopsy can be considered	Tumors <2 cm • Surveillance: G1, low G2, asymptomatic, mainly in the head, no radiological signs suspicious for malignancy, patient factors • Surgery: G2, symptoms, patient wishes Tumors >2 cm • Surgery • Limited resection only if conditions favorable to preserve organ function (otherwise, oncological resection)	EUS, MRI (or CT) every 6 to 12 mo • No change: surveillance • Increase in size (>0.5 cm) or final diameter >2 cm: surgery
NANETS 2020	Pancreatic protocol CT, MRI is also useful Somatostatin receptor–PET imaging should replace ^{111}In-pentetreotide scanning.	EUS-FNA should be performed in patients where making the diagnosis of a PNET would be helpful, or when there is a question about tumor grade.	It is recommended that the decision to observe or resect an asymptomatic PNET 1 to 2 cm in size be individualized. Criteria that should be considered in decision making include age and comorbidities, tumor growth over time, estimated risk of symptom development, details of imaging, grade, the extent of surgical resection required, the patient's wishes, and access to long-term follow-up.	Initial observation without a plan for immediate surgical resection is an acceptable treatment strategy for asymptomatic patients with pancreatic tumors smaller than 1 cm in size and with imaging characteristics consistent with a PNET. In such patients, biopsy is not routinely necessary to confirm the diagnosis before making a decision for observation.

	Screening: Imaging	Screening: Biochemistry	Indication for Surgery	Surveillance
NCCN 2022	Recommended: CT or MRI. As appropriate: SSTR-PET/CT or SSTR-PET/MRI EUS	–	Small (≤2 cm) • Observation in select cases: Observation can be considered for small (≤2 cm), low-grade, incidentally discovered, nonfunctioning tumors. Decision based on estimated surgical risk, site of tumor, and patient comorbidities. • Enucleation or resection ± regional lymphadenectomy Larger (>2 cm), invasive, or node-positive tumors • Resection ± regional lymphadenectomy	12 wk to 12 mo: • History and physical examination • Biochemical markers as clinically indicated • CT/MRI • SSR-based imaging and FDG-PET/CT scan are not recommended for routine surveillance >1 to 10 y: Every 6 mo: • History and physical examination • Biochemical markers as clinically indicated • CT/MRI • SSR-based imaging and FDG-PET/CT scan are not recommended for routine surveillance
MEN1-Related NF-PNET	**Screening: Imaging**	**Screening: Biochemistry**	**Indication for Surgery**	**Surveillance**
MEN1 practice guidelines 2012	Recommended modalities: MRI, CT or EUS. Recommended frequency: yearly	Recommended yearly CgA, PP and glucagon.	Consider surgery for tumors that are more than 1 cm in size and/or show significant growth over 6 to 12 mo.	Similar to screening
MEN1 consensus statement 2020	Recommended modalities: MRI and if available EUS. Consider SSTR-PET/CT or SSTR-PET/MRI for staging if a PNET is detected.	CgA, PP and glucagon are not of added value for the diagnosis of NF-PNETs.	Surgery is recommended for NF-PNETs >2 cm, those with progression under surveillance and grade 2 tumors.	Recommended modalities: MRI or EUS. Consider SSTR-PET/CT or SSTR-PET/MRI for staging. Recommended frequency: individualized based on growth rate.

(continued on next page)

Table 2
(continued)

MEN1-Related NF-PNET	Screening: Imaging	Screening: Biochemistry	Indication for Surgery	Surveillance
ENETS 2016	Recommended modalities: MRI and EUS. SSTR-PET-CT or SSTR-PET-MRI are recommended for staging but not for screening.	No specific recommendation for MEN1.	Routine surgical exploration not generally recommended for PNETs ≤2 cm or NF-PNETs on imaging studies. In patients with PNETs >2 cm, enucleation/local resection at surgery is possible in many patients, whereas pancreatoduodenectomy is reserved for specific selected cases. For patients under surveillance surgical exploration is recommended if there is an increase in size of >0.5 mm or size reaches >2 cm. In addition, surgical exploration is recommended in grade 2 tumors.	Similar to sporadic NF-PNET.
NANETS 2020	Not specifically covered. It is stated that EUS should be performed in patients with MEN1 to identify multifocal disease	None	NF-PNETs smaller than 1 cm can be observed, whereas tumors larger than 2 cm should generally be resected. For tumors between 1 and 2 cm, this should be individualized on additional factors such as grade if available, growth rate, family history, patient factors and symptoms.	Not discussed.

| NCCN 2022 | Recommended modalities are: CT or MRI and as appropriate EUS or SSTR-PET/CT Recommended frequency: Every 1 to 3 y | On clinical indication only | Tumors larger than 2 cm in size. Tumors with relatively rapid rate of growth over 6 to 12 mo. | Recommended modalities are CT, MRI or serial EUS with a preference for studies without radiation for long-term follow-up. Recommended frequency: every 1 to 3 y. |

Abbreviations: CgA, Chromogranin A; CT, Computed Tomography; ENETS, European Neuroendocrine Tumor Society; EUS, Endoscopic Ultrasound; MEN1, multiple endocrine neoplasia type 1; MRI, Magnetic Resonance Imaging; NANETS, North American Neuroendocrine Tumor Society; NCCN, National Comprehensive Cancer Network; NF, nonfunctioning; PNET, pancreatic neuroendocrine tumor; PP, pancreatic polypeptide; SSTR-PET/CT, somatostatin-receptor positron emission tomography/computed tomography.

Data from Falconi et al., ENETS Consensus Guidelines Update for the Management of Patients with Functional Pancreatic Neuroendocrine Tumors and Non-Functional Pancreatic Neuroendocrine Tumors, Neuroendocrinology 2016[10]; Howe et al., The North American Neuroendocrine Tumor Society Consensus Paper on the Surgical Management of Pancreatic Neuroendocrine Tumors, Pancreas 2020[9]; Halfdanarson et al., The North American Neuroendocrine Tumor Society Consensus Guidelines for Surveillance and Medical Management of Pancreatic Neuroendocrine Tumors, Pancreas 2020[2]; Shah et al., NCCN Guidelines Version 1.2022 Neuroendocrine and Adrenal Tumors[11]; Thakker et al., Clinical Practice guidelines for MEN1, Journal of Clinical Endocrinology and Metabolism 2012[8]. Niederle et al. Multiple Endocrine Neoplasia Type 1 and the Pancreas: Diagnosis and Treatment of Functioning and Nonfunctioning Pancreatic and Duodenal Neuroendocrine Neoplasia within the MEN1 Syndrome—An International Consensus Statement, Neuroendocrinology 2021.[12]

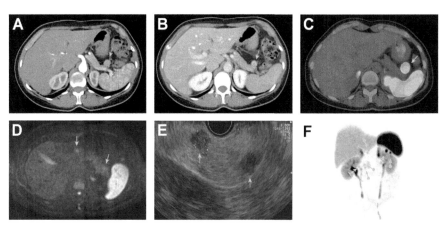

Fig. 2. Imaging of sporadic and MEN1-related nonfunctioning PNETs. Patient 1 with a sporadic nonfunctioning pancreatic neuroendocrine tumor of 1.7 cm in the pancreatic tail (*A*). Arterial phase CT showing a 17 mm pancreatic neuroendocrine tumor (*B*). Portovenous phase CT of the same tumor (*C*). 68Ga-labeled SSTR-PET showing the pancreatic neuroendocrine tumor. Patient 2 with MEN1 (*D*). MRI diffusion weighted imaging showing two subcentimeter pancreatic neuroendocrine tumors (*E*). Endoscopic ultrasound showing two subcentimeter pancreatic neuroendocrine tumors (*F*). 68Ga-labeled SSTR-PET showing multiple pancreatic (*circle* and *arrow*) and duodenal (*line* and *arrow*) neuroendocrine tumors. The arrows indicate the nonfunctioning pancreatic neuroendocrine tumor in **Fig 2**A-E. With thanks to Arthur J.A.T. Braat, MD PhD nuclear medicine physician and Leon MG Moons MD PhD, gastroenterologist for providing the images.

surveillance for NF-PNETs <2 cm is a viable treatment strategy at least for mid-term follow-up. During active surveillance, tumor growth was observed in 22% to 24%, metastases were not seen in tumors <2 cm, and resections were performed in 12% to 14% of patients, mainly because of tumor growth or patient preference.[16,17] Most of the included studies were retrospective, single-center studies, had limited sample size and different inclusion criteria (such as tumor sizes up to 4 cm). Hence the systematic reviews observed considerable heterogeneity between studies, and possible publication bias.

In a recent retrospective multicenter study several of these limitations were overcome by using strict criteria for active surveillance including asymptomatic <2 cm NF-PNETs without radiological signs of malignancy in patients willing to undergo active surveillance.[18] After propensity score matching, none of the patients in the active surveillance (radiological follow-up every 6 months) or upfront resection group died of disease. The estimated overall survival was similar and estimated excess death risk was near zero in both groups.[18] One prospective multicenter study assessed an active surveillance strategy in 76 patients with a mean NF-PNET size of 1.2 cm. Eight (11%) patients had tumor progression >0.5 cm/y, six (8%) underwent resection and no PNET-related deaths were observed during a median follow-up of 17 months (interquartile range 8 to 35 months).[19] These data indicate that active surveillance is an oncologically safe alternative for most patients with an NF-PNET <2 cm. Nevertheless, active surveillance demands access to long-term follow-up, and may perpetuate cancer fear in patients. Three studies show that in clinical practice a significant number of patients with NF-PNETs <2 cm undergo resection. In German and US multicenter studies 29.2% and 44.5% of all patients with a PNET undergoing resection had a tumor <2 cm.[20,21] In a single center study from Italy including 110

Table 3
Characteristics and outcomes of systematic reviews on surveillance for sporadic nonfunctioning pancreatic neuroendocrine tumors

Author (Ref.), Year	No. Included Studies	No. Included Patients	Tumor Size	Growth	Secondary Surgery	Reasons for Resection	Metastases (%)	Survival (%)	Median f/u (Months)
Sallinen,[9] 2017	6[a]	344[b]	10 to 14 mm (range 3 to 33 mm)	84/267 (31%) range across studies 0% to 51%, pooled estimate 22% ([95% CI 7% to 41%], I^2 = 89%)	49/332 (15%) pooled estimate 12%, ([95% CI 4% to 23%], I^2 = 83%)	Cannot be extracted	0 (0%)	NR	32 to 45
Partelli,[10] 2017	5	327[c]	NR	74/312 (23.7%) Range across studies 0% to 51%	46 patients (14.1%)	Tumor size increase (n = 19), patient preference (n = 18), physician preference (n = 7), appearance of symptoms (n = 1) and pancreatic duct dilatation (n = 1)	3/327 (0.9%)[d]	No disease related deaths	28 to 45

Abbreviations: CI, confidence interval; f/u, follow-up; NR, not reported.
[a] 6 studies including patients with sporadic PNET and 3 studies including MEN1-related PNET.
[b] 344 patients with sporadic PNET and another 64 with MEN1-related PNET.
[c] 540 included of which 327 in active surveillance group.
[d] All three patients in one study with distant metastases had NF-PNETs larger than 2 cm.

patients with NF-PNET <2 cm, 73 (72%) underwent surveillance whereas 28 (28%) underwent upfront resection.[22] Reasons for upfront surgery in this study echo recommendations from the guidelines: patient preference (32%), a young age (14.5%), taking into consideration the need for long-term follow-up, and G2 tumors (14.5%) for which risk of (distant) metastases is higher. In addition, the presence of strong positivity at 18F-fluoro-2-deoxyglucose (^{18}F-FDG) PET (21.5%) and the presence of main pancreatic duct (MPD) dilatation (17.5%) were also reason for upfront surgery.[22] In patients with resected NF-PNETs <2 cm on cross-sectional imaging, biliary or MPD dilatation were associated with recurrence.[23] The prognostic value of [18]FDG PT/CT is discussed below. In line with these observations, the NANETS guidelines conclude that individual surgeons are capable of selecting patients with NF-PNETs <2 cm who will potentially benefit from surgical resection although there is no uniform endorsement of surgical resection in such patients.[9]

Surveillance strategy: frequency and modality
ENETS and NCCN guidelines propose an active surveillance strategy with imaging as the cornerstone. Biochemical markers are of limited use in the surveillance of NF-PNETs. Regarding radiological follow-up, the ENETS guidelines suggest MRI or EUS every 6 to 12 months.[10] The NCCN guidelines recommend an initial CT or MRI at 12 weeks to 12 months and every 6 to 12 months thereafter.[11] Early repeat imaging 3 to 6 months after diagnosis can be used to identify rapidly growing tumors that likely are not suitable for active surveillance. MRI should be considered over CT to minimize the radiation risk. Based on the results of cross-sectional imaging SSTR-PET/CT could be additionally performed.

Prognostic factors to guide management
Accepted criteria to guide clinical management for NF-PNETs are tumor size and WHO grade. Tumor size is the most readily available prognostic factor and the agreement between the radiological and pathologic tumor size is high.[24] In patients undergoing resection, larger size is related to malignancy, tumor grade, lymph node metastases, and survival. Of patients with tumors <2 cm 18.9% were deemed to have the malignant disease compared with 85.4% of those with tumors >4 cm.[25]

WHO grade is likely the strongest predictor of survival.[26] Preoperatively WHO grade can be obtained through EUS-guided FNA, although this can both overestimate and underestimate WHO grade since tumor size and intra-tumoral heterogeneity affect the accuracy of EUS-FNA in predicting tumor grade. In a recent meta-analysis, the pooled estimated concordance rate between EUS and surgical grading based on Ki-67 was 80% (95% CI 76-85).[27] Undergrading was significantly more frequent than overgrading.[27] Although WHO grade is useful in predicting the postoperative oncological prognosis, its role in patient selection for operative resection or active surveillance is less well-established. Even among patients with NF-PNETs G1 <2 cm who are eligible for active surveillance instead of upfront surgery, lymph node metastases are found. A large systematic review ($n = 13,374$) found weighted median rates of lymph node metastases of 11.2% in tumors <2 cm and 10.3% in G1 NF-PNETs.[28] Lymph node metastases were associated with worse recurrence-free and overall survival.[28] It should be kept in mind that these numbers are for patients with NF-PNETs <2 cm who were referred for resection, thereby representing a selected population.

Hence, additional prognostic factors are needed for small NF-PNETs that enable personalized decision-making for active surveillance versus upfront surgery as well as when to intervene during active surveillance. Promising in this regard are novel tissue and blood-based biomarkers, which are discussed below.

Tissue-based factors

Novel tissue-based factors that may guide management are (epi)genetic tumor characteristics. The most common genetic alterations in PNETs are seen in the *MEN1* gene, alpha-thalassemia/mental retardation X-linked (*ATRX*) and death domain-associated protein 6 (*DAXX*) genes and the mTOR pathway, whereas alterations in chromatic remodeling genes and *CDKN2A* occur in lower frequencies (**Table 4**). In addition, PNETs often show chromosomal losses and gains in chromosomes 1, 2, 3, 6, 10, 11, 16 and 22.[29,30]

Somatic alternations in *ATRX/DAXX,* which occur in 40% of PNETs and are mutually exclusive[31], are in particular very promising prognostic biomarkers for NF-PNETs (**Fig. 3**). Loss of function of either of these two proteins leads in 85% to telomere dysfunction resulting in general genomic instability and alternative lengthening of telomeres (ALT).[32,33] Both ATRX/DAXX alterations and ALT are strong predictors for NF-PNET-related metastases and are negatively correlated with disease-free survival.[34] This also holds true for NF-PNETs <2 cm.[35] Loss of immunolabeling for DAXX or ATRX is correlated with mutations in their corresponding genes[36,37] and both ATRX/DAXX and ALT can reliably be assessed on biopsies using immunochemistry and fluorescence in situ hybridization, respectively.[38] This allows preoperative assessment of these biomarkers in NF-PNETs, which may enable recognition of high-risk small NF-PNETs. No prospective or comparative studies have been performed to date, therefore ATRX/DAXX nor ALT are not yet regularly used to guide clinical management. Nonetheless, the recently updated 2022 WHO classification of neuroendocrine neoplasms recommends routine determination of ATRX/DAXX and/or ALT status at pathologic examination of NF-PNETs for prognostic purposes.[39]

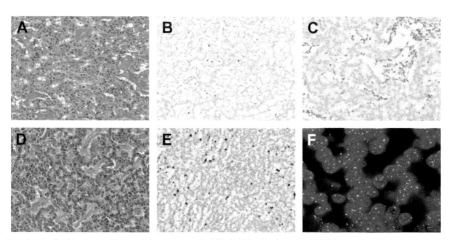

Fig. 3. Pathologic analysis of two sporadic NF-PNETs. Patient 1: H&E immunochemistry (IHC) showing pancreatic neuroendocrine tumor morphology (*A*), Ki-67 IHC of <2% corresponding with grade 1 (*B*) and loss of ATRX on IHC (*C*). Patient 2: H&E IHC showing pancreatic neuroendocrine tumor morphology (*D*), Ki-67 IHC of 10% to 15% corresponding with grade 2 (*E*) and presence of Alternative Lengthening of Telomeres on Fluorescence In Situ Hybridization (*F*).

Table 4
Frequently altered genes in sporadic nonfunctional pancreatic neuroendocrine tumors

Genetic Alteration	Incidence in (NF-)PNETs Measured by:		Biologic Role and Role in NF-PNET Tumorigenesis	Prognostic Value	Prospective Validation
	Genomic Alteration	Immunohistochemistry			
MEN1	44% sporadic mutations (Sanger Sequencing)[31]	25.3% to 50% loss of nuclear staining.[81,82]	MEN1 gene is located on the 11q13 locus. Its product, menin, is a nuclear protein involved in the regulation of gene transcription by coordinating chromatin remodeling. MEN1 mutations are usually an early event in NF-PNET tumorigenesis.	• Loss of MEN1 is associated with higher WHO tumor grade, larger tumor size, liver metastasis, hormone production, and vascular invasion.[82] • Loss of MEN1 is not shown to have an association with recurrence or metastasis.[82]	N/A
ATRX/DAXX	43% (Sanger Sequencing)[31]	25% loss of nuclear staining.[35]	ATRX and DAXX genes are located on the Xq21.1 and 6p21.32 chromosome, respectively. The products of these genes, interact with one another and play multiple cellular roles, including chromatin remodeling at telomeres where they regulate the deposition of histone variant H3.3 during the assembly of pericentromeric and telomeric chromatin. ATRX/DAXX mutations are mutually exclusive and usually a late event in NF-PNET tumorigenesis. Mutations in ATRX/DAXX lead to general chromosomal instability resulting in ALT.	• Both loss of ATRX/DAXX on immunochemistry and/or ALT are independent prognostic biomarkers for RFS in NF-PNETs, including small NF-PNETs (≤2.0 cm).[35]	Not performed

TSC2 (mTOR Pathway)	8.8% (Sanger Sequencing)[31]	53% to 59% loss or low nuclear staining.[82,83]	TSC2 is located on chromosome 16p13.3 and is a tumor suppressor gene that encodes for the protein tuberin. Tuberin interacts with hamartin to form the TSC protein complex. This complex is a negative regulator in the PI3K/Akt/mTOR pathway in which it controls cell growth.	• Loss of TSC2 expression associated with larger tumor size, nodal metastasis, liver metastasis, recurrence, hormone production, and vascular invasion.[82,83] • Loss of TSC2 expression is associated with shorter OS and RFS.[82,83]	Not performed
PTEN (mTOR Pathway)	7.3% (Sanger Sequencing)[31]	25% to 38% loss or low nuclear staining.[82,83]	PTEN gene is located on chromosome 10q23 and is a tumor suppressor gene that promotes cell growth, protein synthesis and transcription. PTEN is a negative regulator of the PI3K/Akt/mTOR pathway its loss facilitates activation of the pathway in cancer cells.	• Loss of PTEN was associated with larger tumor size, recurrence and vascular invasion.[82] • Loss of PTEN was associated with shorter OS and metastatic disease.[82,83]	Not performed
PIK3CA (mTOR Pathway)	1.4% (Sanger Sequencing)[31]	NR	PIK3CA is located on chromosome 3q26.32. Its protein has several cell functions including proliferation and survival. PIK3CA is involved in the mTOR pathway.	• It is not described that mutations in PIK3CA have an association with recurrence or metastasis.	N/A
ARID1A	10% (Next generation sequencing[84] Loss of copy number deletion in 10% of primary PNETs (measured with FISH)[85]	43% loss of expression[86]	ARID1A is located on the 1p36 locus and encodes for the corresponding protein which is chromatin remodeler.	Loss of ARID1A was associated with regional lymph node metastasis, elevated Ki-67 index and neural invasion.[86] Loss of ARID1A is independent predictor of OS.[86]	Not performed

(continued on next page)

Table 4
(continued)

Genetic Alteration	Incidence in (NF-)PNETs Measured by:		Biologic Role and Role in NF-PNET Tumorigenesis	Prognostic Value	Prospective Validation
	Genomic Alteration	Immunohistochemistry			
SETD2	5% (Whole Genome Sequencing)[29,32]	8% loss of H3K36me3[85]	SETD2 is located on the 3p21.31 chromosome. It encodes for a histone methyltransferase that is specific for H3 lysine 36 trimethylation (H3K36me3).	• Either loss or deletion in DAXX, ATRX, H3K36me3, ARID1A and/or CDKN2A associated with larger mean tumor size, higher WHO grade, lymphovascular invasion, higher pathologic tumor stage, synchronous distant metastases and metachronous distant metastases.[85]	Not performed
CDKN2A	0% mutations (Sanger Sequencing)[87] Loss of copy number deletion in 7% of primary PNETs (measured with FISH)[85] Copy number loss in 81% primary PNETs with metastases (Whole-exome sequencing)[85]		CDKN2 is located on chromosome 9q21.3 and encodes for p16(INK4A) and the p14(ARF) proteins. CDKN2A is a tumorsupressor gene due to its role in the cell cycle regulation.	• Either loss or deletion in DAXX, ATRX, H3K36me3, ARID1A and/or CDKN2A was associated with larger mean tumor size, higher WHO grade, lymphovascular invasion, higher pathologic tumor stage, synchronous distant metastases and metachronous distant metastases.[85] • PNETs with either loss or deletion in DAXX, ATRX, H3K36me3, ARID1A and/or CDKN2A had a shorter DFS and DSS.[85]	Not performed

Abbreviations: ARID1A, AT-Rich Interaction Domain 1A; ATRX, alpha-thalassemia/mental retardation X-linked; CDKN2A, Cyclin-dependent kinase inhibitor 2A; DAXX, Death domain-associated protein; DFS, disease free survival; DSS, disease specific survival; MEN1, multiple endocrine neoplasia type-1; NF-PNET, nonfunctioning neuro-endocrine tumor; NR, Not reported; OS, overall survival; PIK3CA, Phosphatidylinositol 3-Kinases; PTEN, phosphate and tensin homolog; RFS, relapse free survival; SETD2, SET domain containing 2; TSC2, tuberous sclerosis 2.

Epigenetic studies identified two main NF-PNET subtypes, resembling either pancreatic α or β cells of the islands of Langerhans expressing transcriptional factors ARX and PDX1, respectively.[39–41] These subtypes show varying degrees of biomarkers associated with disease progression and prognosis. Beta cell-like tumors harbor few genomic alterations and copy number variations (CNVs) and tend to have a low recurrence rate. Alpha cell-like tumors often harbor *MEN1* mutations but differ with regard to presence of *ATRX/DAXX* mutations and CNVs.[39] Alpha-like tumors with *ATRX/DAXX* mutations and/or more extensive CNVs behave more aggressively compared with alpha-like tumors without *ATRX/DAXX* mutations and few CNVs.[39] These epigenetic profiles, combined with mutational and chromosomal copy number alteration data, may be promising tools for the risk-stratification of NF-PNETs.

Blood-based factors

Novel blood-based biomarkers are urgently needed for PNETs. In this regard, multi-analyte assessment of tumor biology is preferred over mono-analyte evaluation of membrane antigens or secretory products.[42] The most promising biomarker is the NETest, a blood-based multi-analyte gene transcription biomarker. A recent meta-analysis showed the NETest to have an 85% accuracy of differentiating stable from progressive disease in sporadic neuroendocrine tumors of different origin.[43] In addition, the NETest anticipated RECIST-defined disease status up to 1 year before imaging in patients with gastroenteropancreatic neuroendocrine tumors.[44] However, outcome data (overall and progression-free survival) based on NETest-guided management are not available yet. In addition, no data is available specifically for its use in small NF-PNETs. Circulating tumor DNA (ctDNA) may be another interesting approach, but presently ctDNA positivity has not been shown in non-metastatic PNETs.

Imaging-based factors

The use of [18]FDG PET was recently evaluated in patients undergoing PET and resection. Although [18]FDG positivity was associated with larger tumor size, G2 tumors and higher Ki-67 values, for NF-PNETs <2 cm [18]FDG positivity was not associated with predictors of recurrence.[45]

Innovative imaging-based prognostication for PNETs is still in the early stages of development, and presently used in research only. For example, MRI features such as apparent and true diffusion coefficients, were inversely correlated to histopathological Ki-67 labeling in one study.[46] Radiomics—a novel method for the quantitative description of medical imaging which extracts disease-related information within images, which is not perceptible with the human eye—is currently being developed for CT and MRI. CT-based radiomic features are associated with tumor grade and survival.[47,48] For MRI, the radiomics field is expanding.[49]

Multiple Endocrine Neoplasia Type 1-Related Nonfunctional Pancreatic Neuroendocrine Tumor

Screening and diagnostic workup

Unless the discovery of a PNET leads to a new MEN1 diagnosis, NF-PNETs in patients with MEN1 are generally diagnosed either on the first pancreatic imaging performed after an MEN1 diagnosis or during prospective screening (**Box 1**).

With regard to biochemical screening, the authors of a recent systematic review on the diagnosis of NF-PNETs in MEN1 made a strong recommendation based on moderate quality evidence that annual biochemical screening for NF-PNET is not recommended, due to the limited diagnostic accuracy of the investigated biomarkers.[50]

Box 1
Case vignettes

Case 1.
A 35-year-old woman is seen at the outpatient clinic. On imaging for other reasons a 12-mm lesion in the pancreatic tail was seen. EUS-guided FNA led to the diagnosis PNET WHO grade 1. There are no signs and symptoms of a functioning tumor and no elevated hormones upon testing. Careful history taking reveals a brother with hypercalcemia and kidney stones at the age of 25. Subsequent genetic testing confirms MEN1. The patient is followed with active surveillance.

Case 2.
A 65-year-old man is seen by the geneticist because his sibling has been diagnosed with MEN1. Genetic testing is positive for the family mutation. He is referred to the endocrinologist and among others MRI pancreas is performed. This reveals a 28-mm cystic PNET in the pancreatic tail, a 9 mm PNET in the uncinate process and three additional subcentimeter lesions in the pancreatic body/tail which are most likely PNETs. No evidence of a functioning tumor. The patient is referred to the endocrine surgeon and an enucleation of the 28-mm cystic PNET is performed. Pathology reveals a pT2 (2.5 cm) WHO grade 1 PNET. A neuroendocrine micro-adenoma is also seen. For the other PNETs the patient is followed with active surveillance by yearly MRI.

Case 3.
A 6-year-old girl is seen by the pediatric endocrinologist because she has a parent with MEN1. At the age of 12 the first MRI abdomen is performed which is normal. Repeat MRI abdomen at the age of 15 reveals three PNETs in the pancreatic tail less than 5 mm. Repeat MRI after 1 year shows stable PNETs. She is followed with active surveillance by yearly MRI.

This recommendation is followed by the NCCN, NANETS and an international consensus statement on MEN1.[2,9,11,12] Hence, imaging is the cornerstone of screening for NF-PNETs in MEN1 (see **Fig. 2**). As a preferred screening modality, the authors of the aforementioned systematic review recommend a combined strategy with MRI and EUS.[50] Although EUS is the most sensitive screening method, disadvantages are its invasiveness, the fact that it is operator dependent and not universally available, its inability to fully assess intra-abdominal metastases and suboptimal sensitivity in the pancreatic tail.[50] Moreover, the clinical relevance of the detection of additional sub-centimeter NF-PNETs is questionable. MRI performs more homogeneous throughout the pancreas, but may miss clinically-relevant NF-PNETs as can occur with EUS.[50] CT is considered the least suitable screening modality given the equal sensitivity compared with MRI and the cumulative risk of exposure to ionizing radiation.[50] SSTR-PET/CT is not recommended for screening in MEN1, but does have a place in staging and during active surveillance.[10,12,50] The size of MEN1-related PNETs can be reliably estimated on preoperative imaging.[51]

Recommendations with regard to the age at which pancreatic screening should be initiated in MEN1 range from 10 to 16 years.[8,52–54] In a recent study by the DutchMEN Study Group (DMSG), the estimated probabilities of having a clinically-relevant NF-PNET was 2.5% at age 13.5 and of 5% at age 17.8, which resulted in the recommendation to initiate screening around the age of 13 to 14 years.[55]

Once a diagnosis of NF-PNET is made in a patient with MEN1, additional workup may be performed depending on the size and characteristics of the tumor. Given the high prior probability of having an NF-PNET and the characteristic appearance on imaging, FNA for diagnosis is not needed unless there is doubt about the diagnosis or there are worrisome features. In tumors >1 cm or when surgery is considered, SSTR-PET/CT can be performed for staging as it is superior to conventional imaging for the detection of lymph node and distant metastases.[50,56,57] In addition, CT may be useful preoperatively to assess anatomy and guide surgical planning. NCCN guidelines recommend performing EUS before surgery to assess and localize tumors.[11]

Surgical indications and active surveillance for nonfunctional pancreatic neuroendocrine tumors <2 cm

The decision to proceed to surgery in MEN1-related NF-PNETs is complex. Usually, there are multiple NF-PNETs, even though there may be one dominant tumor. In addition, there may also be concomitant functioning duodenopancreatic (dp) neuroendocrine tumors (see **Fig. 2**) and other MEN1-related active manifestations. Therefore, these decisions should always be made in a multidisciplinary team. Pancreatic surgery for NF-PNETs in MEN1 is associated with a high rate of complications. In the DMSG cohort of 61 patients who underwent surgery for an NF-PNET, 33% developed a major early complication, 20% developed exocrine pancreatic insufficiency and 13% endocrine pancreatic insufficiency.[58]

The 2012 MEN1 Clinical Practice Guidelines recommend surgical resection for NF-PNETs >1 cm or those smaller that show significant growth.[8] Since the publication of the guidelines, retrospective cohort studies have shown that most NF-PNET <2 cm have an indolent natural course.[59,60] Moreover, retrospective studies comparing surgery with active surveillance for patients with NF-PNETs <2 cm showed excellent outcomes for active surveillance and could not show a benefit on metastases-free survival for upfront surgery.[61,62] However, liver metastases occurred in 3% to 4% of patients during active surveillance.[59–62] Recent guidelines therefore advise surgical resection for MEN1-related NF-PNETs that are >2 cm, show progression under surveillance, and—if that information is available—those with WHO G2 tumors.[2,9,10,12]

Surveillance strategy: frequency and modality

If an active surveillance strategy is followed, imaging remains the cornerstone. There are no reliable biomarkers that can replace imaging. Although the exact role of different imaging modalities in active surveillance needs to be delineated, MRI alone or alternating with EUS is generally recommended.[50] Keeping to one modality increases comparability of investigations. EUS is insufficient on its own as it does not allow the detection of intra-abdominal metastases. EUS should therefore either be performed alternating with MRI or coupled with SSTR-PET/CT. During active surveillance, SSTR-PET/CT can be performed on indication for staging purposes, for example, in growing tumors or in the case of uncertainty about potential metastases on conventional imaging. The frequency of surveillance should be tailored to the growth rate of the NF-PNETs.[12] It is advisable to repeat imaging 6 months after an NF-PNET is diagnosed to assess growth rate. If stable, imaging is performed yearly, and depending on the size and duration of stability intervals might be increased to up to 2 years.[50]

Prognostic factors to guide management

Presently, the only actionable prognostic factors in patients with MEN1-related PNETs are tumor size, tumor growth and tumor grade.[63] MEN1-related NF-PNETs >2 cm are associated with a higher risk of metastases as are G2 tumors.[63] Given the shown indolence of most NF-PNETs <2 cm, progression under surveillance is generally considered an indication for intervention.

Other potential factors that may guide management, but are currently not part of the standard-of-care are germline genotype and novel tissue-, radiology- and blood-based biomarkers. Germline genotype is covered in a separate section of this issue, so we will not go into this here.

Tissue-based factors

Tissue-based factors such as ATRX/DAXX and ALT, sporadic genetic alterations as described in **Table 4** and epigenetic profiles resembling α and β lineage differentiation have only been studied to a limited extent in MEN1. It has been shown that *ATRX/DAXX* mutations, and resulting ALT, indeed occur in MEN1-related PNETs and was mainly observed as a late event, seen only in tumors >3 cm or lymph node metastases.[64] Also ARX and PDX1 expression, as surrogate markers for α-cell and β-cell like PNETs, has been examined in MEN1 patients with functioning and NF tumors.[40] ALT was shown to occur in PNETs expressing ARX or PNETs that were double negative for ARX and PDX1. Relapse occurred only in ARX expressing and ALT positive PNETs. Importantly, ALT positivity was only identified in tumors >2 cm, as were relapses. The presence of *ATRX/DAXX* mutations and ALT, its association with ARX positive PNETs, and its association with relapse is in line with studies in sporadic PNETs and suggest extrapolation of this evidence to MEN1-related PNETs. If and how assessment of ATRX/DAXX or ALT can be used in small MEN1-related NF-PNETs remains to be determined.

Blood-based factors

As in sporadic NF-PNETs, reliable blood-based biomarkers to guide management for individual patients are an unmet need in MEN1. There are no data regarding the NET-est in MEN1. Metabolomics may be another area of biomarker research in MEN1, as recently a 3-marker polyamine signature was identified that distinguished patients with MEN1 with dPNETs metastatic to the liver from patients with MEN1 with or without a dPNET but without distant metastases.[65]

Imaging-based factors

Radiology-based biomarkers are of interest because of their noninvasive character and because patients with MEN1 already adhere to a lifelong radiological screening program. In a small prospective cohort study of 18 patients with MEN1 diagnosed through cascade screening, a lower maximum standardized uptake value on 68-Gallium-Dotatate PET/CT (<12.3) was associated with shorter median progression-free survival.[66] In a retrospective cohort study in the Tasmanian cohort FDG-avidity of PNETs was associated with higher grade and metastases.[67] More data on these features and the potential use of radiomics is needed before this can be implemented in clinical practice.

Nonsurgical interventions in sporadic and multiple endocrine neoplasia type 1-related nonfunctional pancreatic neuroendocrine tumors

Surgical resection is presently the only curative treatment of sporadic and MEN1-related NF-PNETs. Nonsurgical treatment options that would allow early treatment of PNETs without the complications and long-term risks of pancreatic insufficiency associated with surgery could lead to an important paradigm shift in the management of these tumors. Presently, none of the available nonsurgical treatment options are considered standard-of-care or an alternative to surgical resection. They are mainly considered in patients who are unfit for or unwilling to undergo surgery.

Endoscopic ultrasound-guided ablative therapies

EUS-guided ablation with either radiofrequency (RFA) or ethanol (EA) is one of these nonsurgical treatment options for small NF-PNETs. For EUS-RFA, most studies recommend a 5 mm distance to surrounding structures to avoid thermal injuries,

Table 5
Characteristics and outcomes of systematic reviews on endoscopic ultrasound-guided ablative therapies

Author (Ref.), Year	No. Included Studies	No. Included Patients	Mean Tumor Size (mm)	Technical Success[a]	Clinical Success[b]	Overall Adverse Events[c]	Acute Pancreatitis[c]	Months of Follow-Up
Rimbas,[69] 2020 EUS-EA	22	F: 33 (MEN1: 4) NF: 50 (MEN1: 2)	F 13 NF 12.6	—	F 93.9% NF 62.1%	F $n = 12$ NF $n = 11$	F 5/33 NF 8/50	F mean 13.5 NF mean 17.0
Garg[68] 2022 EUS-EA[d]	7	91	12.2 ± 1.7	96.7% (90.8 to 98.8)	82.2% (95% CI 68.2 to 90.8)	11.5% (95% CI 4.7 to 25.4)	7.6% (95% CI 3.8 to 14.6)	1 to 60
Rimbas[69] 2020 EUS-RFA	13	F: 25 (MEN1: 1) NF: 44 (MEN1: 3)	F 14.3 NF 16.5	—	F 96% NF 82.4%	F $n = 1$ NF $n = 9$	F: 0 NF: $n = 4$	F mean 9.5 NF mean 13.3
Garg[68] 2022 EUS-RFA[e]	13	113	16.4 ± 5.1	94.4% (88.3 to 97.4)	85.2% (95% CI 75.9 to 91.4)	14.1% (95% CI 7.1 to 26.3)	7.8% (95% CI 4.1 to 14.4)	1 to 60

Abbreviations: EA, ethanol ablation; EUS endoscopic ultrasound; F, Functioning; MEN1, Multiple Endocrine Neoplasia Type 1; NF, Nonfunctioning; RFA, radio frequency ablation.
[a] Technical success, defined as the ability to perform the session as planned.
[b] In Rimbas et al. success was defined as disappearance of the symptoms in patients with functioning PNETs (per patient) and radiological evidence of complete tumor ablation in patients with NF-PNETs (per lesion). Garg et al. defined success rate per lesion as resolution of the clinical syndrome or, for NF-PNETs, complete ablation/disappearance or absence of enhanced area within the tumors based on follow-up contrast enhanced imaging.
[c] Rimbas et al. total number of events. Garg et al. rate per session.
[d] In the EUS-RFA studies 42% of the lesions was functioning.
[e] In the EUS-EA studies 38% of the lesions was functioning.

indicating that RFA cannot be safely applied to all tumors. Recently a review (2020) and a meta-analysis (2022) on this topic have been published.[68,69] Most patients included in these studies were either unable or unwilling to undergo surgery. Results have been summarized in **Table 5**. In the meta-analysis clinical success rates were approximately 80% and 86% and not different between EUS-RFA and EUS-EA.[68] The adverse event rate was between 10% and 15% per session, also not significantly different between the two ablative techniques.[68] Long-term outcomes were not reported in this review. In the review from 2020 results were reported separately for functioning and NF-PNETs, showing a lower success rate for NF-PNETs.[69] Only the 2020 review mentioned the included patients with MEN1 ($n = 10$), but no separate data were shown. In conclusion, although EUS-guided ablative therapy seems safe and reasonably effective in the short-term with respect to syndrome or lesion control, long-term outcome data are lacking. An important outcome would be the effect on the occurrence of metastases. Specifically for MEN1 the effect on pancreatic function from repetitive treatments of different tumors and the feasibility of surgical resection after EUS-guided ablation would be of interest. No comparative studies of EUS-guided RFA or EA versus operative resection or active surveillance have been conducted. Such data are warranted before the exact role of EUS-guided ablation for small NF-PNETs can be determined.

Magnetic resonance imaging-guided radiotherapy
Another local therapy that is of interest for both sporadic and MEN1-related PNETs is MRI-guided radiotherapy using the 1.5 T MR-guided linear accelerator (MR-Linac).[70] There are no data on its use in PNETs. At this time, the Dutch PRIME study (NCT05037461), a single-arm interventional cohort study in patients with MEN1, is recruiting. The study aims to assess efficacy and safety of MRI-guided radiotherapy for the treatment of PNETs in MEN1. Expected completion date is January 1, 2024.

Chemoprevention
Finally, another area of active research mainly in patients with MEN1, is that of chemoprevention with somatostatin analogues (SSA) such as lanreotide. As SSA have proven anti-proliferative effect in advanced PNETs[71,72], the question has been raised if SSA may be used as chemoprevention in small MEN1-related NF-PNET with the ultimate goal to prevent metastatic disease. Animal studies in mouse models of *MEN1* PNET have shown the ability of SSA to decrease tumor proliferation.[73–75] One small non-controlled retrospective study assessed the effect of first-line SSA on MEN1-related PNETs <2 cm with a treatment duration of 12 to 72 months.[76] In this study 80% of the patients had stable disease, 10% had progression and 10% had an objective tumor response.[76] In a small non-controlled prospective study, eight patients with MEN1-related PNETs received first-line SSA during 24 months and were observed up until 72 months.[77] All patients had stable disease in terms of tumor size.[77] Recently, an observational cohort study compared lanreotide with active surveillance in 42 patients with MEN1 and one or more PNETs <2 cm.[78] Patients were free to choose for lanreotide treatment and the median follow-up was 6 years.[78] There was improved RECIST progression-free survival in the lanreotide group.[78] In both groups however, one patient developed liver metastases.[78] Although promising, evidence is insufficient to recommend the use of SSA in small NF-PNETs in MEN1 and prospective randomized trials are needed.

As patients with MEN1 are at known high-risk for the development of NF-PNETs and are often diagnosed before they develop NF-PNETs, novel preventative treatments are a potential high-impact area of future research.

SUMMARY

The incidence of small NF-PNET is increasing. Imaging is the cornerstone of the diagnostic workup, with CT and MRI as the basis. EUS can be added to enable FNA for histologic confirmation of the diagnosis if needed. SSTR-PET is recommended for staging in all patients. Patients with MEN1, who are at high risk for the development of NF-PNETs, are advised to adhere to a life-long imaging-based screening program with MRI and/or EUS. For patients with sporadic, asymptomatic, G1 NF-PNETs <2 cm, initial active surveillance is a safe alternative to surgical resection on a group level; however, identifying the individual patient with a small NF-PNET that potentially benefits from early surgical resection needs improvement. For patients with MEN1 an active surveillance strategy is usually followed until NF-PNETs reach 2 cm in size. In both sporadic and MEN1-related NF-PNETs the most important and clinically-actionable prognostic factors to guide management are tumor size, tumor growth, and tumor grade (WHO). There is an urgent need for novel prognostic factors for small sporadic and MEN1-related NF-PNETs that will enable personalized decision-making for active surveillance or upfront surgery as well as when to intervene during active surveillance. ATRX/DAXX and ALT are promising novel tissue-based markers in this regard. At present nonsurgical treatment options for small NF-PNETs (such as EUS-guided EA or RFA or chemoprevention using somatostatin analogs) are not yet considered an alternative to surgery. They are mainly used for those patients unfit for surgery or unwilling to undergo surgery.

For both sporadic and MEN1-related small NF-PNETs important future directives are the identification of novel prognostic biomarkers enabling accurate and personalized risk stratification and the further development of alternative therapies to surgery. The development of preventative strategies for MEN1-related NF-PNET is of particular interest.

CLINICS CARE POINTS

- Anatomic (CT/MRI/EUS) and molecular (SSTR-PET) imaging have a pivotal role in the diagnosis, staging, and active surveillance of sporadic and MEN1-related NF-PNET.
- Biochemical markers, such as chromogranin A, are not useful in the diagnosis and surveillance of small NF-PNETs.
- The unique challenges in patients with MEN1 arise from the multifocality of both functioning and nonfunctioning dPNETs. In addition, detection differs from sporadic NF-PNETs as patients with MEN1 are screened.
- Surgical resection is recommended for sporadic and MEN-related NF-PNET >2 cm in surgically fit patients.
- Active surveillance is a viable alternative to surgery for sporadic asymptomatic G1 NF-PNETs <2 cm; however, in a small subset of this group high-risk tumors may be present that benefit from upfront resection.
- For patients with MEN1 and NF-PNET an active surveillance strategy is usually followed until a size of 2 cm. Grade 2 tumors provide an indication for upfront surgery in smaller tumors.
- If an active surveillance strategy is chosen, the interval for repeat imaging should be 3 to 6 months and every 6 to 12 months thereafter in sporadic tumors. In MEN1-related tumors, the initial interval is 6 months and yearly thereafter, with considerations of lengthening the interval if tumors show long-term stability.

- Significant increases in size during surveillance, or reaching the threshold of 2 cm are indications for surgical resection both in MEN1-related and sporadic NF-PNETs.
- Novel prognostic factors enabling accurate and personalized risk stratification for patients with NF-PNETs <2 cm are an unmet need.
- 2022 WHO classification of neuroendocrine neoplasms recommends routine determination of ATRX/DAXX and/or ALT status at pathologic examination of NF-PNETs for prognostic purposes.
- Nonsurgical treatment options for NF-PNETs <2 cm are not considered standard-of-care.

DISCLOSURE

The authors have nothing to disclose.

REFERENCES

1. Dasari A, Shen C, Halperin D, et al. Trends in the Incidence, Prevalence, and Survival Outcomes in Patients With Neuroendocrine Tumors in the United States. JAMA Oncol 2017;3(10):1335–42.
2. Halfdanarson TR, Strosberg JR, Tang L, et al. The North American neuroendocrine tumor society consensus guidelines for surveillance and medical management of pancreatic neuroendocrine tumors. Pancreas 2020;49(7):863–81.
3. Lloyd RV, Osamura RY, Kloppel G, et al, editors. WHO classification of tumours of endocrine organs. 4th edition. Lyon: IARC; 2017.
4. Chandrasekharappa SC, Guru S, Manickam P, et al. Positional cloning of the gene for multiple endocrine neoplasia-type 1. Science 1997;276:404–7.
5. Romanet P, Mohamed A, Giraud S, et al. UMD-MEN1 database: an overview of the 370 MEN1 variants present in 1676 patients from the french population. J Clin Endocrinol Metab 2019;104(3):753–64.
6. de Laat JM, van der Luijt RB, Pieterman CR, et al. MEN1 redefined, a clinical comparison of mutation-positive and mutation-negative patients. BMC Med 2016;14(1):182.
7. Goudet P, Murat A, Binquet C, et al. Risk factors and causes of death in MEN1 disease. A GTE (Groupe d'Etude des Tumeurs Endocrines) cohort study among 758 patients. World J Surg 2010;34(2):249–55.
8. Thakker RV, Newey PJ, Walls GV, et al. Clinical practice guidelines for multiple endocrine neoplasia type 1 (MEN1). J Clin Endocrinol Metab 2012;97(9):2990–3011.
9. Howe JR, Merchant NB, Conrad C, et al. The North American neuroendocrine tumor society consensus paper on the surgical management of pancreatic neuroendocrine tumors. Pancreas 2020;49(1):1–33.
10. Falconi M, Eriksson B, Kaltsas G, et al. ENETS consensus guidelines update for the management of patients with functional pancreatic neuroendocrine tumors and non-functional pancreatic neuroendocrine tumors. Neuroendocrinology 2016;103(2):153–71.
11. Guidelines. NCCN Guidelines Version 1.2022 Neuroendocrine Tumors of the Pancreas (Well-Differentiated Grade 1/2). National Comprehensive Cancer Network (NCCN). 2022. Accessed. https://www.nccn.org/guidelines/guidelines-detail?category=1&id=1448.
12. Niederle B, Selberherr A, Bartsch DK, et al. Multiple endocrine neoplasia type 1 and the pancreas: diagnosis and treatment of functioning and nonfunctioning

pancreatic and duodenal neuroendocrine neoplasia within the men1 syndrome - an international consensus statement. Neuroendocrinology 2021;111(7):609–30.

13. Refardt J, Hofland J, Wild D, et al. Molecular Imaging of Neuroendocrine Neoplasms. J Clin Endocrinol Metab 2022;107(7):e2662–70.

14. Ambrosini V, Kunikowska J, Baudin E, et al. Consensus on molecular imaging and theranostics in neuroendocrine neoplasms. Eur J Cancer 2021;146:56–73.

15. van Beek DJ, Takkenkamp TJ, Wong-Lun-Hing EM, et al. Risk factors for complications after surgery for pancreatic neuroendocrine tumors. Surgery 2022;172(1): 127–36.

16. Sallinen V, Le Large TY, Galeev S, et al. Surveillance strategy for small asymptomatic non-functional pancreatic neuroendocrine tumors - a systematic review and meta-analysis. HPB (Oxford) 2017;19(4):310–20.

17. Partelli S, Cirocchi R, Crippa S, et al. Systematic review of active surveillance versus surgical management of asymptomatic small nonfunctioning pancreatic neuroendocrine neoplasms. Br J Surg 2017;104(1):34–41.

18. Ricci C, Partelli S, Landoni L, et al. Survival after active surveillance versus upfront surgery for incidental small pancreatic neuroendocrine tumours. Br J Surg 2022;109(8):733–8.

19. Heidsma CM, Engelsman AF, van Dieren S, et al. Watchful waiting for small nonfunctional pancreatic neuroendocrine tumours: nationwide prospective cohort study (PANDORA). Br J Surg 2021;108(8):888–91.

20. Mintziras I, Keck T, Werner J, et al. Implementation of Current ENETS Guidelines for Surgery of Small (</=2 cm) Pancreatic Neuroendocrine Neoplasms in the German Surgical Community: An Analysis of the Prospective DGAV StuDoQ|Pancreas Registry. World J Surg 2019;43(1):175–82.

21. Lopez-Aguiar AG, Ethun CG, Zaidi MY, et al. The conundrum of < 2-cm pancreatic neuroendocrine tumors: A preoperative risk score to predict lymph node metastases and guide surgical management. Surgery 2019;166(1):15–21.

22. Partelli S, Mazza M, Andreasi V, et al. Management of small asymptomatic nonfunctioning pancreatic neuroendocrine tumors: Limitations to apply guidelines into real life. Surgery 2019;166(2):157–63.

23. Sallinen VJ, Le Large TYS, Tieftrunk E, et al. Prognosis of sporadic resected small (</=2 cm) nonfunctional pancreatic neuroendocrine tumors - a multi-institutional study. HPB (Oxford) 2018;20(3):251–9.

24. Paiella S, Impellizzeri H, Zanolin E, et al. Comparison of imaging-based and pathological dimensions in pancreatic neuroendocrine tumors. World J Gastroenterol 2017;23(17):3092–8.

25. Bettini R, Partelli S, Boninsegna L, et al. Tumor size correlates with malignancy in nonfunctioning pancreatic endocrine tumor. Surgery 2011;150(1):75–82.

26. Rindi G, Klersy C, Albarello L, et al. Competitive Testing of the WHO 2010 versus the WHO 2017 Grading of Pancreatic Neuroendocrine Neoplasms: Data from a Large International Cohort Study. Neuroendocrinology 2018;107(4):375–86.

27. Tacelli M, Bina N, Crino SF, et al. Reliability of preoperative pancreatic neuroendocrine tumors grading on endoscopic ultrasound specimens: a systematic review with meta-analysis of aggregate and individual data. Gastrointest Endosc 2022;S0016-5107(22):01831–4.

28. Tanaka M, Heckler M, Mihaljevic AL, et al. Systematic review and metaanalysis of lymph node metastases of resected pancreatic neuroendocrine tumors. Ann Surg Oncol 2021;28(3):1614–24.

29. Hong X, Qiao S, Li F, et al. Whole-genome sequencing reveals distinct genetic bases for insulinomas and non-functional pancreatic neuroendocrine tumours: leading to a new classification system. Gut 2020;69(5):877–87.
30. Parilla M, Chapel D, Hechtman JF, et al. Recurrent loss of heterozygosity in pancreatic neuroendocrine tumors. Am J Surg Pathol 2022;46(6):823–31.
31. Jiao Y, Shi C, Edil BH, et al. DAXX/ATRX, MEN1, and mTOR pathway genes are frequently altered in pancreatic neuroendocrine tumors. Science 2011; 331(6021):1199–203.
32. Scarpa A, Chang DK, Nones K, et al. Whole-genome landscape of pancreatic neuroendocrine tumours. Nature 2017;543(7643):65–71.
33. Clynes D, Jelinska C, Xella B, et al. Suppression of the alternative lengthening of telomere pathway by the chromatin remodelling factor ATRX. Nat Commun 2015; 6:7538.
34. Wang F, Xu X, Ye Z, et al. Prognostic significance of altered ATRX/DAXX gene in pancreatic neuroendocrine tumors: a meta-analysis. Front Endocrinol (Lausanne) 2021;12:691557.
35. Hackeng WM, Brosens LAA, Kim JY, et al. Non-functional pancreatic neuroendocrine tumours: ATRX/DAXX and alternative lengthening of telomeres (ALT) are prognostically independent from ARX/PDX1 expression and tumour size. Gut 2022;71(5):961–73.
36. Marinoni I, Kurrer AS, Vassella E, et al. Loss of DAXX and ATRX are associated with chromosome instability and reduced survival of patients with pancreatic neuroendocrine tumors. Gastroenterology 2014;146(2):453–60, e455.
37. Singhi AD, Liu TC, Roncaioli JL, et al. Alternative lengthening of telomeres and loss of DAXX/ATRX Expression predicts metastatic disease and poor survival in patients with pancreatic neuroendocrine tumors. Clin Cancer Res 2017;23(2): 600–9.
38. Hackeng WM, Morsink FHM, Moons LMG, et al. Assessment of ARX expression, a novel biomarker for metastatic risk in pancreatic neuroendocrine tumors, in endoscopic ultrasound fine-needle aspiration. Diagn Cytopathol 2020;48(4): 308–15.
39. Rindi G, Mete O, Uccella S, et al. Overview of the 2022 WHO Classification of Neuroendocrine Neoplasms. Endocr Pathol 2022;33(1):115–54.
40. Cejas P, Drier Y, Dreijerink KMA, et al. Enhancer signatures stratify and predict outcomes of non-functional pancreatic neuroendocrine tumors. Nat Med 2019; 25(8):1260–5.
41. Dreijerink KM, Hackeng WM, Singhi AD, et al. Clinical implications of cell-of-origin epigenetic characteristics in non-functional pancreatic neuroendocrine tumors. J Pathol 2022;256(2):143–8.
42. Oberg K, Modlin IM, De Herder W, et al. Consensus on biomarkers for neuroendocrine tumour disease. Lancet Oncol 2015;16(9):e435–46.
43. Öberg K, Califano A, Strosberg JR, et al. A meta-analysis of the accuracy of a neuroendocrine tumor mRNA genomic biomarker (NETest) in blood. Ann Oncol 2020;31(2):202–12.
44. van Treijen MJC, van der Zee D, Heeres BC, et al. Blood molecular genomic analysis predicts the disease course of gastroenteropancreatic neuroendocrine tumor patients: a validation study of the predictive value of the NETest. Neuroendocrinology 2021;111(6):586–98.
45. Paiella S, Landoni L, Tebaldi S, et al. Dual-tracer (68Ga-DOTATOC and 18F-FDG-)-PET/CT scan and G1-G2 nonfunctioning pancreatic neuroendocrine tumors: a

single-center retrospective evaluation of 124 nonmetastatic resected cases. Neuroendocrinology 2022;112(2):143–52.

46. Lotfalizadeh E, Ronot M, Wagner M, et al. Prediction of pancreatic neuroendocrine tumour grade with MR imaging features: added value of diffusion-weighted imaging. Eur Radiol 2017;27(4):1748–59.

47. Liang W, Yang P, Huang R, et al. A combined nomogram model to preoperatively predict histologic grade in pancreatic neuroendocrine tumors. Clin Cancer Res 2019;25(2):584–94.

48. Luo Y, Chen X, Chen J, et al. Preoperative prediction of pancreatic neuroendocrine neoplasms grading based on enhanced computed tomography imaging: validation of deep learning with a convolutional neural network. Neuroendocrinology 2020;110(5):338–50.

49. Bezzi C, Mapelli P, Presotto L, et al. Radiomics in pancreatic neuroendocrine tumors: methodological issues and clinical significance. Eur J Nucl Med Mol Imaging 2021;48(12):4002–15.

50. van Treijen MJC, van Beek DJ, van Leeuwaarde RS, et al. Diagnosing nonfunctional pancreatic NETs in MEN1: The Evidence Base. J Endocr Soc 2018;2(9):1067–88.

51. van Beek DJ, Verkooijen HM, Nell S, et al. Reliability and Agreement of Radiological and Pathological Tumor Size in Patients with Multiple Endocrine Neoplasia Type 1-Related Pancreatic Neuroendocrine Tumors: Results from a Population-Based Cohort. Neuroendocrinology 2021;111(8):705–17.

52. Manoharan J, Raue F, Lopez CL, et al. Is Routine Screening of Young Asymptomatic MEN1 Patients Necessary? World J Surg 2017;41(8):2026–32.

53. Herath M, Parameswaran V, Thompson M, et al. Paediatric and young adult manifestations and outcomes of multiple endocrine neoplasia type 1. Clin Endocrinol (Oxf) 2019;91(5):633–8.

54. Goudet P, Dalac A, Le Bras M, et al. MEN1 disease occurring before 21 years old: a 160-patient cohort study from the Groupe d'etude des Tumeurs Endocrines. J Clin Endocrinol Metab 2015;100(4):1568–77.

55. Klein Haneveld MJ, van Treijen MJC, Pieterman CRC, et al. Initiating pancreatic neuroendocrine tumour (pNET) screening in young MEN1 patients: results from the DutchMEN Study Group. J Clin Endocrinol Metab 2021;106(12):3515–25.

56. Mennetrey C, Le Bras M, Bando-Delaunay A, et al. Value of Somatostatin Receptor PET/CT in Patients With MEN1 at Various Stages of Their Disease. J Clin Endocrinol Metab 2022;107(5):e2056–64.

57. Cuthbertson DJ, Barriuso J, Lamarca A, et al. The Impact of (68)Gallium DOTA PET/CT in Managing Patients With Sporadic and Familial Pancreatic Neuroendocrine Tumours. Front Endocrinol (Lausanne) 2021;12:654975.

58. Nell S, Borel Rinkes IHM, Verkooijen HM, et al. Early and Late Complications After Surgery for MEN1-related Nonfunctioning Pancreatic Neuroendocrine Tumors. Ann Surg 2018;267(2):352–6.

59. Triponez F, Sadowski SM, Pattou F, et al. Long-term Follow-up of MEN1 Patients Who Do Not Have Initial Surgery for Small </=2 cm Nonfunctioning Pancreatic Neuroendocrine Tumors, an AFCE and GTE Study: Association Francophone de Chirurgie Endocrinienne & Groupe d'Etude des Tumeurs Endocrines. Ann Surg 2018;268(1):158–64.

60. Pieterman CRC, de Laat JM, Twisk JWR, et al. Long-Term Natural Course of Small Nonfunctional Pancreatic Neuroendocrine Tumors in MEN1-Results From the Dutch MEN1 Study Group. J Clin Endocrinol Metab 2017;102(10):3795–805.

61. Nell S, Verkooijen HM, Pieterman CRC, et al. Management of MEN1 Related Nonfunctioning Pancreatic NETs: A Shifting Paradigm: Results From the Dutch-MEN1 Study Group. Ann Surg 2018;267(6):1155–60.

62. Partelli S, Tamburrino D, Lopez C, et al. Active Surveillance versus Surgery of Nonfunctioning Pancreatic Neuroendocrine Neoplasms </=2 cm in MEN1 Patients. Neuroendocrinology 2016;103(6):779–86.

63. Sadowski SM, Pieterman CRC, Perrier ND, et al. Prognostic factors for the outcome of nonfunctioning pancreatic neuroendocrine tumors in MEN1: a systematic review of literature. Endocrine-related cancer 2020;27(6):R145–61.

64. de Wilde RF, Heaphy CM, Maitra A, et al. Loss of ATRX or DAXX expression and concomitant acquisition of the alternative lengthening of telomeres phenotype are late events in a small subset of MEN-1 syndrome pancreatic neuroendocrine tumors. Mod Pathol 2012;25(7):1033–9.

65. Fahrmann JF, Wasylishen AR, Pieterman CRC, et al. A Blood-based Polyamine Signature Associated With MEN1 Duodenopancreatic Neuroendocrine Tumor Progression. J Clin Endocrinol Metab 2021;106(12):e4969–80.

66. Lastoria S, Marciello F, Faggiano A, et al. Role of (68)Ga-DOTATATE PET/CT in patients with multiple endocrine neoplasia type 1 (MEN1). Endocrine 2016;52(3):488–94.

67. Kornaczewski Jackson ER, Pointon OP, Bohmer R, et al. Utility of FDG-PET Imaging for Risk Stratification of Pancreatic Neuroendocrine Tumors in MEN1. J Clin Endocrinol Metab 2017;102(6):1926–33.

68. Garg R, Mohammed A, Singh A, et al. EUS-guided radiofrequency and ethanol ablation for pancreatic neuroendocrine tumors: A systematic review and meta-analysis. Endosc Ultrasound 2022;11(3):170–85.

69. Rimbaş M, Horumbă M, Rizzatti G, et al. Interventional endoscopic ultrasound for pancreatic neuroendocrine neoplasms. Dig Endosc 2020;32(7):1031–41.

70. Hehakaya C, Sharma AM, van der Voort Van Zijp JRN, et al. Implementation of Magnetic Resonance Imaging-Guided Radiation Therapy in Routine Care: Opportunities and Challenges in the United States. Adv Radiat Oncol 2022;7(5):100953.

71. Caplin ME, Pavel M, Cwikla JB, et al. Lanreotide in metastatic enteropancreatic neuroendocrine tumors. N Engl J Med 2014;371(3):224–33.

72. Caplin ME, Pavel M, Cwikla JB, et al. Anti-tumour effects of lanreotide for pancreatic and intestinal neuroendocrine tumours: the CLARINET open-label extension study. Endocrine-related cancer 2016;23(3):191–9.

73. Lopez CL, Joos B, Bartsch DK, et al. Chemoprevention with Somatuline(c) Delays the Progression of Pancreatic Neuroendocrine Neoplasms in a Mouse Model of Multiple Endocrine Neoplasia Type 1 (MEN1). World J Surg 2019;43(3):831–8.

74. Quinn TJ, Yuan Z, Adem A, et al. Pasireotide (SOM230) is effective for the treatment of pancreatic neuroendocrine tumors (PNETs) in a multiple endocrine neoplasia type 1 (MEN1) conditional knockout mouse model. Surgery 2012;152(6):1068–77.

75. Walls GV, Stevenson M, Soukup BS, et al. Pasireotide Therapy of Multiple Endocrine Neoplasia Type 1-Associated Neuroendocrine Tumors in Female Mice Deleted for an Men1 Allele Improves Survival and Reduces Tumor Progression. Endocrinology 2016;157(5):1789–98.

76. Ramundo V, Del Prete M, Marotta V, et al. Impact of long-acting octreotide in patients with early-stage MEN1-related duodeno-pancreatic neuroendocrine tumours. Clin Endocrinol 2014;80(6):850–5.

77. Cioppi F, Cianferotti L, Masi L, et al. The LARO-MEN1 study: a longitudinal clinical experience with octreotide Long-Acting Release in patients with Multiple Endocrine Neoplasia type 1 Syndrome. Clin cases mineral bone Metab 2017;14(2): 123–30.
78. Faggiano A, Modica R, Lo Calzo F, et al. Lanreotide Therapy vs Active Surveillance in MEN1-Related Pancreatic Neuroendocrine Tumors < 2 Centimeters. J Clin Endocrinol Metab 2020;105(1).
79. Pieterman CRC, Valk GD. Update on the clinical management of multiple endocrine neoplasia type 1. Clin Endocrinol (Oxf) 2022;97(4):409–23.
80. Pieterman CRC, van Leeuwaarde RS, van den Broek MFM, et al. Multiple Endocrine Neoplasia Type 1. In: Feingold KR, Anawalt B, Boyce A, et al, editors. Endotext. South Dartmouth (MA): MDText.com, Inc.Copyright; 2000. © 2000-2022, MDText.com, Inc.
81. Kim HS, Lee HS, Nam KH, et al. p27 Loss is associated with poor prognosis in gastroenteropancreatic neuroendocrine tumors. Cancer Res Treat 2014;46(4): 383–92.
82. Uemura J, Okano K, Oshima M, et al. Immunohistochemically Detected Expression of ATRX, TSC2, and PTEN Predicts Clinical Outcomes in Patients With Grade 1 and 2 Pancreatic Neuroendocrine Tumors. Ann Surg 2021;274(6):e949–56.
83. Missiaglia E, Dalai I, Barbi S, et al. Pancreatic endocrine tumors: expression profiling evidences a role for AKT-mTOR pathway. J Clin Oncol 2010;28(2): 245–55.
84. Puccini A, Poorman K, Salem ME, et al. Comprehensive Genomic Profiling of Gastroenteropancreatic Neuroendocrine Neoplasms (GEP-NENs). Clin Cancer Res 2020;26(22):5943–51.
85. Roy S, LaFramboise WA, Liu TC, et al. Loss of chromatin-remodeling proteins and/or CDKN2A associates with metastasis of pancreatic neuroendocrine tumors and reduced patient survival times. Gastroenterology 2018;154(8):2060–2063 e2068.
86. Han X, Chen W, Chen P, et al. Aberration of ARID1A Is Associated With the Tumorigenesis and Prognosis of Sporadic Nonfunctional Pancreatic Neuroendocrine Tumors. Pancreas 2020;49(4):514–23.
87. Yachida S, Vakiani E, White CM, et al. Small cell and large cell neuroendocrine carcinomas of the pancreas are genetically similar and distinct from well-differentiated pancreatic neuroendocrine tumors. Am J Surg Pathol 2012;36(2): 173–84.

Lobectomy or Total Thyroidectomy—Where Is the Pendulum now for Differentiated Thyroid Cancer?

Oliver J. Fackelmayer, MD[a,b,]*, William B. Inabnet III, MD, MHA[a,c]

KEYWORDS

- Differentiated thyroid cancer • Lobectomy • Thyroidectomy • Extent of surgery
- Complications • Recurrence • Completion

KEY POINTS

- Low-risk differentiated thyroid cancers can be adequately and appropriately treated with thyroid lobectomy.
- Thyroid lobectomy is associated with fewer adverse events compared with total thyroidectomy, even for experienced high-volume surgeons.
- Thyroid lobectomy can avoid the need for thyroid hormone supplementation.
- Preoperative risk assessment rests on thorough sonographic evaluation and patient selection.
- Be prepared to convert a planned thyroid lobectomy to total thyroidectomy with central lymph node dissection if intraoperative findings necessitate.
- Completion thyroidectomy may be required for previously unsuspected high-risk histology or findings on final pathologic condition.
- Perioperative risk assessment should complement anticipated dynamic surveillance with extent of surgery decision-making.

INTRODUCTION

Differentiated thyroid cancers include papillary thyroid carcinoma and follicular thyroid carcinoma. Papillary thyroid carcinoma is by far the most common type of thyroid cancer, accounting for more than 85% of cases. Poorly differentiated thyroid carcinoma,

[a] Divsion of General, Endocrine and Metabolic Surgery, University of Kentucky, Lexington, KY 40508, USA; [b] General, Endocrine & Metabolic Surgery, University of Kentucky, 125 East Maxwell Street, Suite 302, Lexington, KY 40508, USA; [c] Department of Surgery, University of Kentucky College of Medicine, UK HealthCare, 800 Rose Street, MN268, Lexington, KY 40508, USA
* Corresponding author. General, Endocrine & Metabolic Surgery, University of Kentucky, 125 East Maxwell Street, Suite 302, Lexington, KY 40508.
E-mail address: oliver.fackelmayer@uky.edu

Surg Oncol Clin N Am 32 (2023) 373–381
https://doi.org/10.1016/j.soc.2022.10.011
1055-3207/23/© 2022 Elsevier Inc. All rights reserved.

Table 1		
Operation nomenclature		
Nomenclature	**Unilateral**	**Bilateral**
Reference term	*Thyroid lobectomy*	*Total thyroidectomy*
Alternative term	*Hemithyroidectomy*	*Near-total thyroidectomy*
Antiquated/ambiguous term	*Partial thyroidectomy*	*Subtotal thyroidectomy*

including anaplastic thyroid cancer, accounts for less than 3% of cases and is not considered in this discussion of initial choice of operation. Finally, medullary thyroid carcinoma is a neuroendocrine-derived tumor and requires a definitive upfront operation beyond the scope discussed here.

The first-line treatment of differentiated (papillary and follicular) thyroid carcinomas is surgery. Historically, a preoperative diagnosis of thyroid cancer mandated a total thyroidectomy, routinely combined with central lymph node dissection, with the associated risk of nerve injury, hypoparathyroidism, and postoperative hematoma. One of the guiding principles for this aggressive upfront surgical approach was the routine use of adjuvant radioactive iodine therapy. A major reworking of the American Thyroid Association Differentiated Thyroid Cancer Guidelines of 2015, there has been a paradigm shift toward a more informed and individualized approach to reign in overtreatment with both excessive extent of index operation and overutilization of radioactive iodine administration.[1,2]

There is confusing nomenclature when discussing thyroid operations (**Table 1**). Partial thyroidectomy and subtotal thyroidectomy are ambiguous and antiquated terms without clear definition and should be avoided. When performing a thyroid operation for known or suspected thyroid cancer, the entire thyroid lobe on the operative side should be removed, leaving as small a cuff of thyroid tissue as possible, if any, at the insertion point of the recurrent laryngeal nerve. In a unilateral operation, the paratracheal visceral compartment is entered on only one side of the central neck. Such an operation is known as a hemithyroidectomy or thyroid lobectomy; we will use thyroid lobectomy as the reference term. A thyroid lobectomy can also include removal of the thyroid isthmus, transection of the isthmus, or preservation of the isthmus. A bilateral operation has been termed a thyroidectomy, near-total thyroidectomy, or total thyroidectomy; we will use total thyroidectomy as the reference term.

Performing the correct operation at initial presentation influences future management of the patient. The goal of the initial thyroid operation is to remove the primary tumor as well as any clinically significant lymph node disease. Here, we will discuss factors to consider when selecting an initial operation, as well as intraoperative findings that may change the planned operation.

PREOPERATIVE DECISION-MAKING

Thyroid cancer is approached based on risk stratification, and that risk is continually restratified with each new piece of data, known as dynamic risk stratification.[3] Preoperatively, risk stratification is both that of the risk of a particular patient undergoing an operation and the risk of thyroid cancer recurrence following that operation.

There are several factors to consider when deciding the extent of the index operation. All patients should undergo a comprehensive history to determine presenting symptoms and history of present illness, past medical history, prior neck surgery, medications, and family history. Voice is assessed both in taking this history and in inquiring as to changes in voice quality. If there is clinical concern for nerve

Table 2
Familial thyroid cancer

Entity:	Gene	Thyroid Cancer Prevalence	Dominant Histologic Subtype	Note
Nonsyndromic familial thyroid cancer	Unknown	22.7%	PTC	3 DTC-affected first-degree relatives
Familial adenomatosis Polyposis	APC	12%	Cribriform-morular variant-PTC	This rare histology subtype should prompt genetic testing for FAP
Cowden syndrome	PTEN	35%	PTC	Also known as PTEN-Hamartoma tumor
Carney complex	PRKAR1A	5%	PTC	
DICER1	DICER1	30%	FTC	
Werner syndrome	WRN	16%	FTC	

Abbreviations: DTC, differentiated thyroid carcinoma; FTC, follicular thyroid carcinoma; PTC, papillary thyroid carcinoma.

involvement from thyroid pathologic condition or prior neck surgery, fiberoptic laryngoscopy to assess vocal cord mobility should be performed.[4] For example, for a patient with prior anterior approach cervical operation, especially if postoperative voice changes, one should ensure normal and symmetric vocal cord mobility with laryngoscopy. Alternatively, transcutaneous laryngeal ultrasound may be adequate in patients with favorable anatomy. A known vocal cord paralysis on the side with pathology would make one hesitant to risk the contralateral nerve if not absolutely necessary. Although 90% of thyroid cancers are sporadic, family history can reveal hereditary thyroid cancer syndromes (**Table 2**).[5] Finally, a history of head and neck radiation or radiation exposure is a significant risk factor for malignancy and total thyroidectomy should be strongly considered.

Mandatory History

- Presenting symptom/HPI (compressive symptoms)
- Prior neck surgery (especially anterior approach spine surgery, prior thyroid, or parathyroid surgery)
- Voice changes (particularly for posteriorly located pathologic condition suspicious for nerve involvement)
- History of head/neck/mediastinal radiation (childhood cancers, Hodgkin lymphoma)
- Radiation exposure, especially during childhood (Chernobyl nuclear accident)
- Family history (thyroid cancer)
- Medications (especially anticoagulation, antiplatelets, and thyroid hormone)

Some patients may come with additional information in the form of somatic genetic mutations such as a nodule with indeterminate cytology (Bethesda III or IV) sent for molecular testing. There are certain mutations, and specifically combinations of mutations, which portend a more aggressive biology and should be considered for total thyroidectomy, such as synchronous BRAF V600 E and TERT promoter mutations.[6] This is an evolving area beyond the scope of discussion in this article.

Preoperative tumor characteristics mandating total thyroidectomy

- Tumor size greater than 4 cm[7]
- Concern for extrathyroidal extension
- Lymph node metastases
- Distant metastatic disease

The ideal patient for thyroid lobectomy is a small, less than 4 cm, differentiated thyroid cancer completely intrathyroidal without evidence of extrathyroidal extension or clinically apparent cervical lymph node metastases. Additionally, the patient should have no history of head and neck radiation, no family history to suggest familial thyroid carcinoma, and not already taking thyroid hormone supplementation.

Sonographic Assessment

The most critical information to guide the appropriateness of thyroid lobectomy is preoperative ultrasound. The tumor is sonographically mapped within the thyroid. An intrathyroidal tumor with a rim of normal thyroid parenchyma on all sides is favorable. A nodule that abuts the thyroid capsule must be particularly scrutinized. If there is capsular distortion (bulging) without evidence of extrathyroidal extension, it can be considered for thyroid lobectomy but close attention must be given intraoperatively for gross extrathyroidal extension with a low threshold for conversion to a total thyroidectomy. The patient should be aware of the risk of requiring a completion thyroidectomy if final pathologic condition demonstrates extrathyroidal extension. Next a detailed sonographic lymph node mapping is performed to assess the central compartment VI and VII lymph nodes, scrutinizing the ipsilateral para tracheal space, pretracheal space (precricoid Delphian lymph nodes and inferior midline lymph nodes), and contralateral paratracheal space. Both the ipsilateral and contralateral lateral neck, compartments II to V should also be thoroughly interrogated. Rounded, enlarged lymph nodes with loss of a normal fatty hilum, hyperechoic foci, and/or cystic change are suspicious and should be biopsied with FNA and thyroglobulin washings or can be sampled at operation for frozen section. In the latter case, the operation should be converted from thyroid lobectomy to total thyroidectomy with compartmental lymph node dissection if positive.

Ultrasound findings favorable for thyroid lobectomy

- Tumor size less than 4 cm
- Intrathyroidal tumor without sonographic evidence of extrathyroidal extension
- No sonographically suspicious lymph nodes
- No contralateral nodules suspicious for multifocal disease

REASONS IN FAVOR OF A UNILATERAL OPERATION (THYROID LOBECTOMY)
TABLE 3
Perioperative Risk Reduction

Inherent to thyroid surgery are certain risks with profound implications for patient outcomes and quality of life. It stands to reason that limiting an operation to one side decreases the perioperative risks.[8] This has been shown to be true even for high volume, experienced thyroid surgeons.[9]

Thyroid Hormone Supplementation

Following a total thyroidectomy, the patient is required to take thyroid hormone replacement indefinitely. Patients, especially younger patients, may be opposed to

Table 3 Pros and cons of thyroid lobectomy	
Thyroid Lobectomy Pros	Thyroid Lobectomy Cons
Perioperative risk reduction	Risk of requiring a second operation for completion thyroidectomy
Potential to avoid thyroid hormone supplementation	Unreliable thyroglobulin monitoring
	Unable to administer radioactive iodine

the idea of being medication-dependent indefinitely. One study, however, has shown that more than 80% of patients following lobectomy for differentiated thyroid cancer will have a TSH greater than 2 and require thyroid hormone supplementation.[10] In addition, lack of access to medication (developing nations or rural areas of the United States) is an important although less common consideration. At least in the short term, quality of life is better following lobectomy compared with total thyroidectomy.[11]

REASONS IN FAVOR OF A BILATERAL OPERATION (TOTAL THYROIDECTOMY) TABLE 4
Avoids the Risk of Requiring a Second Operation (Completion Thyroidectomy)

There are scenarios where a patient would strongly prefer a single operation and would not accept the risk of requiring a completion thyroidectomy. Additionally, some patients with significant perioperative risk factors may benefit from a single definitive operation rather than risking needing a second general anesthetic and perioperative risks.

Tumor Markers for Monitoring Biochemical Recurrence (Thyroglobulin)

Thyroglobulin is a protein made exclusively by thyroid follicular cells and is used as a surrogate tumor marker for thyroid cancer surveillance. Thyroglobulin is trended postoperatively and should be low or undetectable following total thyroidectomy. A low postoperative thyroglobulin can be made even lower following thyroid remnant ablation with radioactive iodine. The thyroglobulin value is difficult to interpret in the presence of thyroglobulin antibodies; however, the antibody level itself can be trended as a marker of recurrence.[12] Additionally, the higher levels present following thyroid lobectomy with a remaining native thyroid lobe are difficult to interpret and trend as the remaining lobe will often hypertrophy.[13] Thus, in cases of thyroid lobectomy for thyroid cancer, surveillance relies even more heavily on ultrasound surveillance for evidence of structural recurrence.

INTRAOPERATIVE DECISION-MAKING

At operation, additional data is available to the surgeon through dissection, inspection, and palpation. Certain findings not expected on preoperative assessment can alter the plan such that a planned thyroid lobectomy should be converted to a total thyroidectomy.

Gross extrathyroidal extension, clinically positive lymph node involvement, or concern for margin involvement are all intraoperative findings that would likely require completion thyroidectomy. If these findings are encountered during surgery, the operation should proceed with total thyroidectomy. Preoperative dedicated ultrasound should have heightened suspicion of these findings before surgery.

Table 4	
Pros and cons of total thyroidectomy	
Total Thyroidectomy Pros	**Total Thyroidectomy Cons**
Single upfront operation (no risk of requiring completion)	Increased upfront operative risk
Thyroglobulin monitoring for biochemical recurrence	Mandatory thyroid hormone replacement
Ability to administer radioactive iodine	

Whenever performing a thyroid lobectomy for a known or suspected malignancy, the patient should be counseled that intraoperative findings could necessitate a total thyroidectomy and the patients should be consented for possible total thyroidectomy with or without central compartment lymph node dissection.

POSTOPERATIVE DECISION-MAKING

Final pathologic condition must be reviewed with a critical eye to ensure an adequate index operation has been achieved. The following findings on final pathologic condition for thyroid lobectomy require completion thyroidectomy be performed to allow for better oncologic surveillance, and in most cases, to administer adjuvant radioactive iodine therapy.

Indications for Completion Thyroidectomy

- Tumor size greater than 4 cm[1,5]
- Consideration for postoperative RAI therapy
- Intermediate risk disease
  - Minor extrathyroidal extension (microscopic ETE)
  - Greater than 5 involved lymph nodes with micrometastatic foci less than 2 mm
  - Vascular invasion
  - Aggressive histology (tall cell, hobnail, cribriform-morular)
- High-risk disease
  - Gross extrathyroidal extension
  - Gross residual disease (incomplete tumor resection)
  - Any involved lymph node that is greater than 3 cm
  - Extranodal extension

Low risk for structural disease recurrence does not require completion thyroidectomy or adjuvant RAI. This includes multifocal papillary thyroid microcarcinoma and micrometastatic lymph node disease (<2 mm) in 5 or fewer nodes.

ONCOLOGIC OUTCOMES

The oncologic treatment goal is to remove all gross disease and minimize the risk of recurrence.

The American Thyroid Association 2015 Guidelines for Adult Patients with Thyroid Nodules and Differentiated Thyroid Cancer has 3 categorical recommendations for the extent of the index operation.[1] These recommendations are all 3 rated strong and supported by moderate-quality evidence.[14–18]

- Total thyroidectomy
  - Primary tumor greater than 4 cm or gross extrathyroidal extension (clinical T4 disease)

○ Clinically apparent lymph node disease (clinical N1) or distant metastatic disease (M1)
- Thyroid lobectomy or total thyroidectomy
  ○ Primary tumor greater than 1 cm and less than 4 cm without extrathyroidal extension and without clinical evidence of lymph nodes metastases (clinical N0).
  ○ The decision is based on treatment team risk assessment and patient preferences.
- Thyroid lobectomy
  ○ Primary tumor less than 1 cm without extrathyroidal extension and without clinical evidence of lymph nodes metastases (clinical N0).
  ○ Additionally, these patients may be candidates for active surveillance.

There has been a mixed adoption of these guidelines.[19–21] However, subsequent analyses with long follow-up have supported thyroid lobectomy for appropriately selected patients with fewer adverse events.[19,22–26]

An important concept when considering outcomes for thyroid surgery is that of salvage for recurrent disease. Whether a patient experiences a recurrence following thyroid lobectomy, or total thyroidectomy, salvage with multimodal therapy is typically possible.[27–29] Multimodal therapy can include reoperation (completion thyroidectomy, recurrence resection, lymph node dissection), with or without adjuvant RAI, salvage RAI without reoperation, or surveillance alone.

SUMMARY

Thyroid lobectomy should be the default operation for properly selected patients with small (<4 cm) low risk (sonographically intrathyroidal without extrathyroidal extension or suspicious lymphadenopathy) differentiated thyroid cancers without a clear indication for total thyroidectomy. Preoperative decision-making with careful sonographic risk assessment is imperative for patient selection. All patients should be counseled on the risk of upgrading the index operation to a total thyroidectomy as well as the risk of requiring a completion thyroidectomy. In addition, the expectation should be set that it is common for patients to require daily thyroid hormone supplementation following thyroid lobectomy. The low rate of recurrence, plus the high likelihood of salvage with multimodal therapy, affords excellent disease-specific survival.

CLINICS CARE POINTS

- Low risk differentiated thyroid cancers can be adequately and appropriately treated with thyroid lobectomy.
- Thyroid lobectomy is associated with fewer adverse events compared to total thyroidectomy, even for experienced high-volume surgeons.
- Thyroid lobectomy can avoid the need for thyroid hormone supplementation. Preoperative risk assessment rests on thorough sonographic evaluation and patient selection.
- Be prepared to convert a planned thyroid lobectomy to total thyroidectomy with central lymph node dissection if intraoperative findings necessitate.
- Completion thyroidectomy may be required for previously unsuspected high-risk histology or findings on final pathology.
- Peri-operative risk assessment should complement anticipated dynamic surveillance with extent of surgery decision-making.

- Perioperative risk assessment should complement anticipated dynamic surveillance with extent of surgery decision-making.

DISCLOSURES/CONFLICT OF INTEREST STATEMENT

The authors have nothing to disclose. No funding sources or financial/commercial conflicts of interest or disclosures related to this study.

REFERENCES

1. Haugen BR, Alexander EK, Bible KC, et al. 2015 American Thyroid Association Management Guidelines for Adult Patients with Thyroid Nodules and Differentiated Thyroid Cancer: The American Thyroid Association Guidelines Task Force on Thyroid Nodules and Differentiated Thyroid Cancer. Thyroid 2016;26(1):1–133.
2. Mayson SE, Chan CM, Haugen BR. Tailoring the approach to radioactive iodine treatment in thyroid cancer. Endocr Relat Cancer 2021;28(10):T125–40.
3. Momesso DP, Vaisman F, Yang SP, et al. Dynamic Risk Stratification in Patients with Differentiated Thyroid Cancer Treated Without Radioactive Iodine. J Clin Endocrinol Metab 2016;101(7):2692–700.
4. Maher DI, Goare S, Forrest E, et al. Routine Preoperative Laryngoscopy for Thyroid Surgery Is Not Necessary Without Risk Factors. Thyroid 2019;29(11):1646–52.
5. Patel KN, Yip L, Lubitz CC, et al. The American Association of Endocrine Surgeons Guidelines for the Definitive Surgical Management of Thyroid Disease in Adults. Ann Surg 2020;271(3):e21–93.
6. Xing M, Liu R, Liu X, et al. BRAF V600E and TERT promoter mutations cooperatively identify the most aggressive papillary thyroid cancer with highest recurrence. J Clin Oncol 2014;32(25):2718–26.
7. Jonklaas J, Sarlis NJ, Litofsky D, et al. Outcomes of patients with differentiated thyroid carcinoma following initial therapy. Thyroid 2006;16(12):1229–42.
8. Fackelmayer OJ, Wu JX, Yeh MW. Endocrine Surgery: Management of Postoperative Complications Following Endocrine Surgery of the Neck. Surg Clin North Am 2021;101(5):767–84.
9. Hauch A, Al-Qurayshi Z, Randolph G, et al. Total thyroidectomy is associated with increased risk of complications for low- and high-volume surgeons. Ann Surg Oncol 2014;21(12):3844–52.
10. Schumm MA, Lechner MG, Shu ML, et al. Frequency of Thyroid Hormone Replacement After Lobectomy for Differentiated Thyroid Cancer. Endocr Pract 2021;27(7):691–7.
11. Chen W, Li J, Peng S, et al. Association of Total Thyroidectomy or Thyroid Lobectomy With the Quality of Life in Patients With Differentiated Thyroid Cancer With Low to Intermediate Risk of Recurrence. JAMA Surg 2022;157(3):200–9.
12. Knappe L, Giovanella L. Life after thyroid cancer: the role of thyroglobulin and thyroglobulin antibodies for postoperative follow-up. Expert Rev Endocrinol Metab 2021;16(6):273–9.
13. Giovanella L, Ceriani L, Garo ML. Is thyroglobulin a reliable biomarker of differentiated thyroid cancer in patients treated by lobectomy? A systematic review and meta-analysis. Clin Chem Lab Med 2022;60(7):1091–100.
14. Matsuzu K, Sugino K, Masudo K, et al. Thyroid lobectomy for papillary thyroid cancer: long-term follow-up study of 1,088 cases. World J Surg 2014;38(1):68–79.

15. Barney BM, Hitchcock YJ, Sharma P, et al. Overall and cause-specific survival for patients undergoing lobectomy, near-total, or total thyroidectomy for differentiated thyroid cancer. Head Neck 2011;33(5):645–9.
16. Mendelsohn AH, Elashoff DA, Abemayor E, et al. Surgery for papillary thyroid carcinoma: is lobectomy enough? Arch Otolaryngol Head Neck Surg 2010;136(11): 1055–61.
17. Haigh PI, Urbach DR, Rotstein LE. Extent of thyroidectomy is not a major determinant of survival in low- or high-risk papillary thyroid cancer. Ann Surg Oncol 2005;12(1):81–9.
18. Nixon IJ, Ganly I, Patel SG, et al. Thyroid lobectomy for treatment of well differentiated intrathyroid malignancy. Surgery 2012;151(4):571–9.
19. Pasqual E, Sosa JA, Chen Y, et al. Trends in the Management of Localized Papillary Thyroid Carcinoma in the United States (2000-2018). Thyroid 2022. https://doi.org/10.1089/thy.2021.0557. published online ahead of print, 2022 Mar 15.
20. McDow AD, Saucke MC, Marka NA, et al. Thyroid Lobectomy for Low-Risk Papillary Thyroid Cancer: A National Survey of Low- and High-Volume Surgeons. Ann Surg Oncol 2021;28(7):3568–75.
21. Puttergill B, Khan S, Christakis I, et al. Thyroid lobectomy for low-risk thyroid cancers. Ann R Coll Surg Engl 2022;104(2):113–6.
22. Song E, Han M, Oh HS, et al. Lobectomy Is Feasible for 1-4 cm Papillary Thyroid Carcinomas: A 10-Year Propensity Score Matched-Pair Analysis on Recurrence. Thyroid 2019;29(1):64–70.
23. Bosset M, Bonjour M, Castellnou S, et al. Long-Term Outcome of Lobectomy for Thyroid Cancer. Eur Thyroid J 2021;10(6):486–94.
24. Bojoga A, Koot A, Bonenkamp J, et al. The Impact of the Extent of Surgery on the Long-Term Outcomes of Patients with Low-Risk Differentiated Non-Medullary Thyroid Cancer: A Systematic Meta-Analysis. J Clin Med 2020;9(7):2316.
25. Kuba S, Yamanouchi K, Hayashida N, et al. Total thyroidectomy versus thyroid lobectomy for papillary thyroid cancer: Comparative analysis after propensity score matching: A multicenter study. Int J Surg 2017;38:143–8.
26. Matsuura D, Yuan A, Harris V, et al. Surgical Management of Low-/Intermediate-Risk Node Negative Thyroid Cancer: A Single-Institution Study Using Propensity Matching Analysis to Compare Thyroid Lobectomy and Total Thyroidectomy. Thyroid 2022;32(1):28–36.
27. Wang LY, Migliacci JC, Tuttle RM, et al. Management and outcome of clinically evident neck recurrence in patients with papillary thyroid cancer. Clin Endocrinol (Oxf) 2017;87(5):566–71.
28. Park JH, Yoon JH. Lobectomy in patients with differentiated thyroid cancer: indications and follow-up. Endocr Relat Cancer 2019;26(7):R381–93.
29. Shokoohi A, Berthelet E, Gill S, et al. Treatment for Recurrent Differentiated Thyroid Cancer: A Canadian Population Based Experience. Cureus 2020;12(2): e7122.

A Nod to the Nodes
An Overview of the Role of Central Neck Dissection in the Management of Papillary Thyroid Carcinoma

Robert Mechera, MD, Dr med habil[a,b,c,*],
Isabella Maréchal-Ross, MD[a], Stan B. Sidhu, PhD, FRACS[a,d],
Peter Campbell, MBBS, FRACS[c], Mark S. Sywak, MMed, FRACS[a,d]

KEYWORDS

- Thyroid cancer • Papillary thyroid cancer • Central neck dissection
- Prophylactic central neck dissection • Recurrence • Micrometastasis • Metastasis

KEY POINTS

- Understanding the central neck anatomy, lymphatic spread, and biological behavior of thyroid cancer is crucial for surgical decision-making regarding the role of central node dissection (CND).
- Selection of patients for a CND is problematic because of the low accuracy of preoperative and intraoperative nodal assessment. Therefore, prophylactic CND (pCND) may be the only reliable method to assess nodal status appropriately.
- Recommendations to perform routine pCND are based on low-level evidence and mainly expert opinion. Obtaining high-level evidence is challenging.
- The effect of pCND on oncological outcomes remains controversial with regard to the reduction of locoregional recurrence, staging, and decision-making for further adjuvant treatment as well as long-term follow-up with thyroglobulin.
- pCND is associated with increased temporary morbidity (hypoparathyroidism, recurrent laryngeal nerve injury), but can be safely performed by experienced surgeons.

[a] Endocrine Surgery Unit, Royal North Shore Hospital, Northern Sydney Local Health District and Northern Clinical School, Sydney Medical School, Faculty of Medicine and Health, University of Sydney, St. Leonards, New South Wales 2065, Australia; [b] Clarunis, University Hospital Basel, Spitalstrasse 21, Basel 4031, Switzerland; [c] Endocrine and Breast Surgery, St. George Hospital, Gray Street, Kogarah, New South Wales 2217, Australia; [d] Sydney Medical School, Faculty of Medicine and Health, University of Sydney, Sydney, New South Wales 2006, Australia
* Corresponding author.
E-mail address: Robert.mechera@gmail.com
Twitter: @RobMechera (R.M.)

Surg Oncol Clin N Am 32 (2023) 383–398
https://doi.org/10.1016/j.soc.2022.10.012
1055-3207/23/© 2022 Elsevier Inc. All rights reserved.

INTRODUCTION

The incidence of thyroid cancer (TC) increased by 20% from 1990 to 2013.[1] The reasons for this development are multifactorial but mainly reflect the higher rate of detecting smaller papillary carcinomas (papillary thyroid cancer, PTC) in particular microcarcinomas (PTMC) (≤ 1 cm).[1,2]

Several prognostic factors, such as age, tumor size, grade, histologic subtype, extrathyroidal extension (ETE), molecular factors ($BRAF^{V600E}$), and distant metastases are well established.[3,4] The association of lymph node metastasis (LNM) and prognosis in well-differentiated TC (WDTC) is, however, less understood. This is reflected by the fact that clinically apparent or microscopic occult regional neck disease is present in 20% to 80% whereas long-term survival remains excellent.[5,6] Although, some studies also showed an increased risk of mortality in younger patients with LNM,[7] the current staging system considers all patients below the age of 55 as stage I disease regardless of their nodal involvement.[8] Hence, LNM is mainly considered a major prognostic factor in older patients.[5,9]

The presence of LNM in PTC, however, is an independent risk factor for the development of locoregional recurrence (LRR).[10] Importantly, characteristics such as clinically evident nodal disease (cN1), larger size (macrometastasis ≥ 2 mm) or the number of metastases as well as extranodal extension are associated with an increased risk of recurrence compared with microscopic disease (micrometastasis <2 mm).[6,11] The American Thyroid Association (ATA) has therefore classified micrometastatic LNM in ≤ 5 nodes as "low risk," greater than 5 metastatic nodes but with <3 cm in size as "intermediate risk" and any LNM >3 cm in size as "high-risk" category for structural disease recurrence.[12]

Therefore, it is generally accepted that a therapeutic compartment-oriented central neck dissection (tCND) in clinically node-positive (cN1) patients has a beneficial impact on both survival and recurrence.[12] However, the long-term effect of prophylactic central neck dissection (pCND) in clinically nodal negative (cN0) patients, harboring mainly microscopic disease, has been an ongoing matter of debate.[12,13]

This review will address the nodal staging, anatomy, and lymphatic drainage in the central compartment and discuss the implication of the extent of surgery. It will further present arguments for and against a routine pCND in PTC based on current literature.

PREOPERATIVE AND INTRAOPERATIVE STAGING OF THE CENTRAL NECK COMPARTMENT
Preoperative

Besides a thorough clinical examination, high-resolution ultrasound (US) has been the mainstay of preoperative nodal staging in PTC and was demonstrated to alter the extent of surgery by 41%.[12,14] The morphologic indicators of nodal involvement are lymph node enlargement, rounded shape, absence of a fatty hilum, irregularity, punctate calcifications, cystic changes, and peripheral vascularity.[15]

The identification of lateral neck disease in the US demonstrated acceptable diagnostic efficacy (sensitivity 70%, specificity 84%).[16] However, imaging of the central neck compartment is more challenging. This is due to the masking presence of the thyroid, frequent micrometastatic disease not detected on imaging, and the location of LNM in the inferior aspect of the neck/superior mediastinum near the air-filled trachea and sternum (sensitivity 33% and specificity of 93%).[15–17]

The presence of malignancy in lymph nodes can further be assessed with US-guided fine-needle aspiration biopsy (FNAB), and if still indeterminate, thyroglobulin (Tg) washings of the needle aspirate.[12] The combination of both increases sensitivity and specificity to almost 100%: Moreover, high titer FNA Tg strongly supports the presence of nodal metastasis.[18] The poor performance of US even in experienced hands in the central compartment means that FNAB of central nodes is rarely performed preoperatively.

With regard to cross-sectional imaging, CT was superior to US to identify abnormal lymph nodes (LN) in regions (superior mediastinum or retropharyngeal region) that are poorly assessable by US (sensitivity: 40% vs 28%).[19] Sensitivity was further improved by a combination of both modalities in comparison to US alone (48% vs 28%).[20] However, the diagnostic accuracy of both US and CT remained unsatisfactory for optimal surgical decision-making and routine CT is generally recommended in advanced disease.[12]

MRI and [18]FDG-PET play a limited role in the initial assessment of LNM in the central neck and are, therefore, not routinely recommended.[12] [18]FDG-PET might be considered when signs of locally advanced disease are present.

Intraoperative

As the prediction of LNM with preoperative imaging is limited, intraoperative visualization, inspection, and palpation by the surgeon is an additional tool to guide operative decision-making regarding CND. However, sensitivity (59%) as well as specificity (67%) of intraoperative determination of central LNM are low.[21]

If the nodal disease is apparent to the surgeon during intraoperative palpation, the frozen section can assist the surgical decision-making, as its diagnostic accuracy is high[22] and the distinction between enlarged nodules in Hashimoto's thyroiditis and LNM is sometimes difficult.[23]

Sentinel LN biopsy in TC using blue dye, radiotracer, or colloid nanoparticles has not gained widespread application because of a low detection rate of around 45% and a high false-negative rate in the range of 20%.[24] This might be explained by the high density of lymphatic vessels, and the growth of the primary tumor into different regions of the thyroid resulting in variability of drainage.[24] Interestingly, some clinicians consider the Delphian node as a sentinel node given its predictive character and advocate for frozen sections as a decision tool for further assessment of the central compartment in cN0 PTC.[25]

Some novel intraoperative diagnostic tools are currently being evaluated. Jonker and colleagues[26] showed a 25% reduction of negative pCNDs with molecular fluorescence-guided imaging and spectroscopy targeting the receptor kinase MET which is overexpressed in PTC[26] This modality will require further evaluation.

ANATOMY OF THE CENTRAL NECK COMPARTMENT

The ATA Surgery working group defined the boundaries of the central neck compartment (levels VI and VII) to enable uniformity of discussions and communication between specialists (**Fig. 1**).[27] The LNs in the central compartment have been grouped into prelaryngeal/Delphian, pretracheal, and right and left paratracheal nodes. Of note, while the left paratracheal nodes are only located anteriorly to the recurrent laryngeal nerve (RLN), the right paratracheal nodes are located anteriorly as well as posteriorly (paraoesophageal) to the RLN (**Fig. 2**).[28–30]

LYMPHATIC DRAINAGE AND PATTERNS OF SPREAD

Lymphatic drainage follows the vasculature of the thyroid, and therefore, metastatic spread usually occurs in a sequential fashion infiltrating first the nodes in the central and later in the lateral neck and superior mediastinum.[28] As such, the lower thyroid

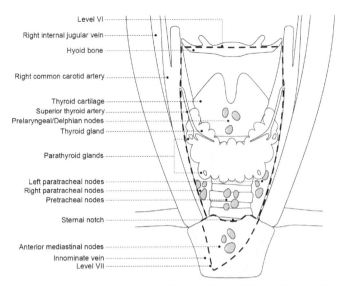

Fig. 1. Anatomy of the central neck (anterior). Boundaries of levels VI and VII: Superior: Hyoid bone; Lateral: Medial borders of the carotid sheaths; Inferior: Innominate artery on the right and corresponding axial plane on the left; Posterior: Deep layer of the deep cervical fascia; Anterior: Superficial layer of the deep cervical fascia.

drains along the inferior thyroid vessels via the paratracheal nodal compartment into the venous angle of the junction between subclavian and internal jugular veins.[31] Drainage of the upper pole, however, follows the superior thyroid vessels toward the jugulodigastric LN and may bypass the central compartment LN.[31] Skip metastases to the lateral neck have been reported in up to 30% of PTC and seem to be more likely in female patients, age greater than 45, small upper pole tumors and vascular invasion.[32–34] Although uncommon, upper pole tumors with aggressive biology can also metastasize to the parapharyngeal nodes.[28,35]

Although unilateral PTCs predominantly spread to the ipsilateral LN basins, isthmic or multifocal PTCs have been shown to metastasize to the central compartment on both sides and occasionally to contralateral lateral nodal basins.[36,37]

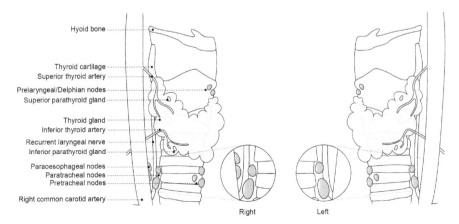

Fig. 2. Anatomy of the central neck (lateral view).

EXTENT OF CENTRAL NECK DISSECTION

A compartment-oriented dissection is preferred over resection of only abnormal LNs.[12,38] This "berry picking" technique is associated with a significantly greater risk of LRR[38] and has been defined in the past as "incomplete surgery."[39]

Based on the ATA statement from 2009,[27] the American Head and Neck Society defined a complete CND as the removal of the prelaryngeal, pretracheal, and paratracheal sub-compartments.[28] It can be either unilateral or bilateral if both paratracheal compartments are resected. Although unilateral dissection can be performed in a therapeutic and prophylactic setting, bilateral CND should be performed more cautiously given the significant morbidity of hypocalcemia and airway compromise due to the risk of bilateral RLN damage.[40] Level VII should be incorporated into every central neck dissection as it is in direct continuity to the pretracheal nodes in level VI and failure to do so could leave the macrometastatic disease behind.[41] However, the extent of the dissection should be adjusted based on the surgeon's assessment of procedural safety.[12]

Some nodal sub-compartments have gained additional importance. First, the prelaryngeal/Delphian LNs should routinely be included in a CND as metastatic involvement is frequent and predictive of LNM in other locations.[25,42,43] Second, the right paraoesophageal nodes are often overlooked and an independent predictor of residual/recurrent disease (see **Fig. 2**).[29,30] Last, thymectomy during CND is not recommended due to minimal oncological benefit and high risk of hypocalcemia because of the frequent intrathymic localization of the inferior parathyroid glands.[44]

LYMPH NODE YIELD

In contrast to other human cancer entities, an optimal nodal yield in PTC has not been clearly defined. Robinson and colleagues[45] estimated that patients falsely staged nodal negative in 53% when only one node was examined, whereas this number decreased to less than 10% when more than six nodes were analyzed.[45] For patients undergoing pCND with T1b, T2, and T3 tumors, 3, 4, and 8 nodes would need to be examined to rule out occult LNM with 90% confidence.[45] In our experience, an adequate unilateral CND should yield a minimum of four lymph nodes.

PROPHYLACTIC NECK DISSECTION
Impact of Prophylactic Central Node Dissection on Locoregional Recurrence

The controversial role of routine pCND in managing TC is reflected in conflicting data which argue both for[46–48] and against[49–53] the use of this approach (**Table 1**).

Reduction of locoregional recurrence with prophylactic central node dissection
Two recent meta-analyses compared patients who underwent total thyroidectomy with (T + pCND) and without pCND (T-pCND) and identified an absolute risk reduction of 1.3% to 2.07% when pCND was performed.[47,48] The impact of pCND on lateral neck recurrence rate was not significantly different.[48]

However, these results need to be interpreted with an understanding of the limitations of the available data:

1. The included studies are mainly retrospective, observational, have significant methodological limitations, and might suffer from migration bias (Will-Rogers Phenomenon).
2. The reduced recurrence rate in the T + pCND group can also be attributed to confounding factors. Patients with pN1 nodal stage are more likely to receive

Table 1
Arguments for and against the performance of prophylactic central neck dissection

For	Against
LNM is common	LNM is mainly micrometastatic and clinical significance is debatable
Reduces the rate of LRR	Evidence regarding the reduction of LRR is conflicting and based on low-level data
pCND might be the only reliable method to assess nodal status due to inaccurate preoperative and intraoperative assessment	LNM is mainly micrometastatic
Reduces re-operative surgery	Re-operative surgery can be safely performed by experienced surgeons
Improves the accuracy of staging and allows a better selection of patients for RAI ablation	Upstaging leads to overtreatment with RAI resulting in RAI-related morbidity
Improves postoperative surveillance with Tg	Tg levels become comparable after RAI ablation and long-term athyroglobulinaemia is common even without RAI ablation
Can be safely performed by experienced surgeons	Increases morbidity for the marginal benefit and most of patients are treated by low-volume surgeons

Abbreviations: LNM, lymph node metastasis; LRR, locoregional recurrence; pCND, prophylactic central neck dissection; Tg, Thyroglobulin.

radioactive iodine (RAI) ablation and more stringent thyroid-stimulating hormone suppression.[47]

No reduction of locoregional recurrence with prophylactic central node dissection

Most of recent studies endorse the lack of an oncological benefit of pCND.[49–52] Two recent meta-analyses included randomized controlled trials (RCT) to assess the effectiveness of pCND and found no significant impact on the structural/biochemical recurrence rate.[49,51] Interestingly, 500 pCNDs were necessary to prevent one recurrence (NNT 500). The main limitation of this meta-analysis was the difference in follow-up times and inclusion criteria.[49,51]

In summary, the outlined data regarding the impact of pCND on LRR are conflicting. In combination with the generally low median rate of recurrence in cN0 PTC at around 2%, a clear statement regarding the improvement of LRR rates after pCND remains problematic.[28,54]

Impact on Staging and Adjuvant Radioactive Iodine Ablation

Proponents of routine pCND argue that the information obtained from the central neck specimen can inform the decision of whether to proceed to RAI ablation through refinement of staging.[12,55,56] As such, patients with central LNM may be upstaged from a pN0 to a pN1a.[8] Moreover, Nylén and colleagues[55] demonstrated that 23% of patients were upgraded into a higher ATA risk category (from "low risk" to" intermediate risk"). In addition, central LNM was an independent factor for recommending RAI ablation with a trend toward higher doses of I-131.[55] In contrast, RAI ablation was more frequently avoided and dosing reduced in patients staged pN0 following pCND.[55]

The information obtained from pCND can play an even larger role when applying the current ATA guidelines where the number and size of metastatic LNs are crucial for adequate risk stratification.[12]

This Approach Faces Significant Criticism

1. There is currently no high-level evidence about the efficacy of RAI ablation in micro-metastatic disease to support a more aggressive administration of RAI.[57]
2. RAI ablation showed no consistent reduction of recurrence, overall survival, or mortality in early-stage PTC.[57]
3. Upstaging can lead to overtreatment with RAI and can cause significant morbidity and reduced quality of life.[58]
4. The rates of clinically relevant upstaging vary significantly across different studies.[56,59]
5. Only patients greater than 55 will be upstaged and consequently offered RAI ablation.[8] However, the indication for RAI ablation varies between centers around the world and adjuvant treatment might be offered based on the presence of LNM alone.[60]

Impact of Prophylactic Central Node Dissection on Surveillance with Thyroglobulin

Another benefit of pCND is the potentially improved surveillance with Tg as a marker of persistent and recurrent disease. Reducing the burden of the disease by pCND has been demonstrated to reduce postoperative Tg levels.[61] However, this effect might only be valid in the early postoperative period, since Tg levels become comparable after RAI ablation and patients without RAI treatment might become athyroglobulinaemic regardless of pCND.[62] Our clinical impression is that pCND is associated with a more thorough clearance of disease from the central compartment with lower postoperative Tg levels.

Impact of Prophylactic Central Node Dissection on Re-operative Surgery

Some authors argue that pCND at the time of initial surgery reduces re-operations, thereby, avoiding challenging re-operations in the central compartment.[63] Moreover, re-operative surgery is less likely to achieve a biochemical cure which might require further interventions. Hence, one can argue that all diseases should be removed during the initial procedure. Although re-operative surgery of the central neck can be safely performed by experienced surgeons, the first procedure is always the best opportunity to achieve a surgical cure.[64]

Morbidity

It is important to carefully balance the advantages of pCND against any added risks. Injury to the RLN and devascularization of the parathyroid glands are major concerns during CND because of their proximity to the paratracheal LNs.[65] Hence, temporary (tempHPT) and permanent hypoparathyroidism (permHPT) (OR 2.23-2-28 and 1.84–2.22, respectively), as well as temporary vocal cord palsy (1.53–2.03), are the common complications of CND.[47,48] Interestingly, one group argues that for every case of LRR potentially prevented, 15 patients may risk permHPT.[51]

Conversely, it has been demonstrated that high-volume surgeons can add CND to a total thyroidectomy without additional risk of morbidity.[50,53,61,66] Although tempHPT can occur at high rates of up to 30% even in experienced hands, the incidence of permanent hypoparathyroidism remained low.[61,66] This effect has been attributed to the liberal use of parathyroid auto-transplantation and routine calcium and vitamin D replacement.[61,66]

Patient Selection for Prophylactic Central Neck Dissection

Current guidelines

There is a strong consensus across all identified national and international guidelines to perform therapeutic neck dissection to remove the structural disease.[12,28,60,67–69] With regard to the recommendation of pCND they, however, differ (**Table 2**).

The 2015 ATA guidelines[12] recommend pCND in advanced tumors with T3 and T4 staging and in patients with clinically involved lateral neck nodes (cN1b). Additionally, pCND can be performed if the information gained will be helpful to plan further steps in the therapy. Based on moderate-level evidence omitting pCND in T1 and T2 cancers is strongly recommended.

Some guidelines go a step further and specify the patient cohort which may profit from pCND further in detail. The American Head and Neck Society[28] follows the ATA guidelines but adds age, multifocality, and ETE to the characteristics that may require pCND. Moreover, a multidisciplinary approach to weighing up risks against benefits on an individual level is encouraged.

The European Society of Endocrine Surgeons (ESES)[70] even recommends routine unilateral pCND in patients with cN1b, T3, and T4 tumors, age $\geq$ 45 or $\leq$ 15 years, male sex, and bilateral or multifocal tumors. It also stresses the fact that pCND should be limited to experienced surgeons.

According to the European Society for Medical Oncology (ESMO),[60] pCND may additionally be performed in some patients with T1 and T2. However, they acknowledge that adherence to their guidelines might vary from center to center.

The recommendation of the 2016 United Kingdom National Multidisciplinary Guidelines finds a more conservative approach. Although pCND is only explicitly recommended in a cN1b situation, pCND in patients with high-risk features (T3 and T4, age $\geq$ 45), multifocality, and suspected ETE should be discussed in the "spirit of personalized decision-making." At the same time, pCND is not recommended if patients have all the following characteristics: Classical PTC, age $\leq$ 45, unifocality, size <4 cm or no ETE on US.

In a further step of de-escalation, the 2022 National Comprehensive Cancer Network (NCCN) guidelines state that pCND in PTC is only indicated in patients with clinically involved lateral nodes (cN1b) but should otherwise not be routinely performed.[68]

In contrast, the Japanese Association of Endocrine Surgeons advocates for a more aggressive approach and generally recommends pCND for all patients with PTC. A certain subset of high-risk patients was not further specified.[69]

Clinicopathological risk factors for central lymph node metastasis

Several clinicopathological risk factors for the development of central LNM have been discussed. Ma and colleagues[71] associated age less than 45, male sex, multifocality, tumor size >1 cm, tumor location in the upper third, lymphovascular invasion, certain histologic high-risk subtypes, capsular invasion, ETE, and BRAF[v600m] mutation with central LNM. Although the relevance of some factors (eg, age, bilaterality, or BRAF[v600m] mutation) varies across different studies and some of them are not available preoperatively, clinicopathological characteristics are fundamental tools to justify treatment intensification and assist the surgeon to decide if a pCND should be performed.

Generating High-Level Evidence

Studies that addressed the topic of pCND mainly derived from low-level data and expert consensus (**Box 1**). Therefore, recommendations are formulated vaguely. Carling and colleagues[72] estimated that an RCT would require the enrollment of 5840

Table 2
Summary of current guidelines on prophylactic neck dissection in papillary thyroid cancer

Guideline/Consensus group	Year	Recommendation	Strength of recommendation/Evidence Level
American Thyroid Association[12]	2015	Ipsilateral or bilateral pCND should be *considered* in • Advanced primary disease T3 and T4 • Clinically involved lateral neck nodes (cN1b) • If the information will be used to plan further steps in therapy	Weak recommendation/ low-quality evidence
American Head and Neck Society[28]	2016	pCND *may* be performed in patients with • T3 and T4 tumors • Older or very young age • Multifocality • ETE • Clinically involved lateral neck nodes (cN1b) • If the information will be used to plan further steps in therapy	Not mentioned
European Society of Endocrine Surgeons (ESES)[70]	2013	*Routine* unilateral pCND in patients: • T3 and T4 tumors • Patients aged ≥ 45 or ≤15 y • Male patients • Bilateral or multifocal tumors • Clinically involved lateral neck nodes (cN1b)	Not mentioned
European Society for Medical Oncology (ESMO)[60]	2016	pCND *may* be performed in T1 and T2 with radiation exposure or family history of TC or aggressive features on cytology or multifocality or suspected ETE • T3, T4 tumors • To be performed in specialized centers	IV C: Optional recommendation level (insufficient evidence for efficacy or benefit does not outweigh the risk or the disadvantages/based on retrospective data)
United Kingdom Multidisciplinary Guidelines[67,83]	2016	• pCND is *recommended* in clinically involved lateral neck nodes (cN1b) • pCND *may* be performed in high-risk tumors (T3 and T4, ≥ 45, multifocality, suspected ETE • Indication should follow personalized decision-making	Not mentioned

(continued on next page)

Table 2 (continued)			
Guideline/Consensus group	Year	Recommendation	Strength of recommendation/Evidence Level
National Comprehensive Cancer Network (NCCN)[68]	2022	• pCND *not* routinely recommended •Only *recommended* in clinically involved lateral neck nodes (cN1b)	2A: Uniform consensus/ based on lower-level evidence
Japanese Association of Endocrine Surgeons[69]	2020	• pCND is *routinely recommended* in the surgery of PTC	Weak recommendation/ poor evidence but good expert consensus

Abbreviations: ETE, extrathyroidal extension; pCND, prophylactic neck dissection.

patients over 7 years to achieve an 80% statistical power.[72] Moreover, the cost for this trial would exceed $20 million and was therefore considered not feasible.[72] Hence, the question that needs to be raised is if the oncological benefits of pCND justify the conduct of such a trial.

Ramirez and colleagues[13] recently assessed the methodological quality of 12 systematic reviews and meta-analyses. Only four studies adhered to methodological standards and all studies have been classified to be of "critically low" methodological quality.[13] They concluded that results based on these recommendations should be used with caution.[13]

The French ESTIMABL3 trial, including 1000 patients with low-risk TC, is planned to terminate in 2026 and might give some further insight into the potential benefits of pCND.

Special Situations

Prophylactic central neck dissection prophylactic central node dissection for patients with papillary microcarcinomas
Although frequent, most of these cancer show indolent behavior and active surveillance has emerged as a valid option to manage a select group of these patients.[2] Nevertheless, there is a subset of patients with PTMC who display a more aggressive behavior with early metastasis and LN involvement.[73,74] A recent meta-analysis identified male gender, multifocality, tumor size greater than 5 mm, and ETE as reliable clinical predictors of central LNM.[75] Although pCND can be considered in these cases, dedicated trials so far failed to demonstrate any oncological benefit.[76]

Prophylactic central neck dissection in patients with cN1b
There is a strong consensus among current guidelines to advocate for a simultaneous pCND when lateral nodes are clinically involved (cN1b).[12,28,67,68,70] However, previous retrospective studies and one meta-analysis have challenged this recommendation and demonstrated that the rate of LRR in the central neck appears to be low, even if patients had the cN1b disease.[77–80] Given the typical pattern of spread of lymph node disease from the thyroid gland to central, and then, lateral compartments, it seems intuitive to clear the ipsilateral levels VI and VII zones in conjunction with a formal lateral lymph node dissection.

Prophylactic central neck dissection in patients with follicular or Hürthle cell cancer.

Follicular (FTC) metastasis is usually hematogenous.[12] However, the presence of cervical LNM usually ranges between 2% and 8% but can reach 17% in widely

> **Box 1**
> **Challenges of current evidence and future trials**
>
> - Recommendations/Consensus mainly based on
>   - Retrospective observational data
>   - Low Quality Systematic Reviews and meta-analyses
>   - Expert consensus
> - Current RCTs Underpowered (low Rate of Structural Recurrence and Surgical Complication)
> - Migration bias (Will-Rogers phenomenon) in studies showing the beneficial impact of pCND
> - High cost, long follow-up, and high number of patients required to conduct a well-powered RCT

invasive FTC and 17% to 34% in HCC.[81,82] Moreover, LNM in FTC seems to be associated with increased mortality.[9] Nevertheless, the role of pCND in FTC and HCC has not been sufficiently addressed and is therefore currently not indicated for patients with FTC.[12,68,69] In contrast, patients with Hürthle cell cancer (HCC) demonstrate LNM in up to 34% of cases.[82] Our preference, therefore, is to approach HCC similarly to papillary thyroid carcinoma and include pCND with thyroidectomy.

SUMMARY

LNM in the central neck in PTC is common but the biological behavior of occult micrometastatic disease and resulting management in cN0 PTC with pCND remains controversial. Based on low-level evidence, international guidelines and consensus statements currently recommend pCND mainly in advanced tumors but the decision to add pCND to the thyroidectomy is more complex and should follow a more individualized approach.

Besides considering clinicopathological risk factors, the endocrine surgeon needs to be familiar with the nature of the disease, surgical techniques, potential benefits, and risks of the procedure. Moreover, surgeons require knowledge about their operative outcomes and complication rates to be able to make a patient-oriented decision if pCND is indicated as CND can be associated with significant morbidity.

With all these factors considered, we continue to employ a routine pCND for papillary thyroid cancers greater than 10 mm, employing careful surgical techniques to preserve RLN function in conjunction with neuromonitoring and liberal use of parathyroid auto-transplantation. We believe that pCND should be an integral component in the modern treatment of TC when undertaken by experienced endocrine surgeons.

DISCLOSURE

The authors have nothing to disclose.

REFERENCES

1. Kim J, Gosnell JE, Roman SA. Geographic influences in the global rise of thyroid cancer. Nat Rev Endocrinol 2020;16(1):17–29.

2. Sugitani I, Ito Y, Takeuchi D, et al. Indications and Strategy for Active Surveillance of Adult Low-Risk Papillary Thyroid Microcarcinoma: Consensus Statements from the Japan Association of Endocrine Surgery Task Force on Management for Papillary Thyroid Microcarcinoma. Thyroid 2021;31(2):183–92.

3. Gillanders SL, O'Neill JP. Prognostic markers in well differentiated papillary and follicular thyroid cancer (WDTC). Eur J Surg Oncol 2018;44(3):286–96.

4. Zhang Z, Zhang X, Yin Y, et al. Integrating BRAF(V600E) mutation, ultrasonic and clinicopathologic characteristics for predicting the risk of cervical central lymph node metastasis in papillary thyroid carcinoma. BMC Cancer 2022;22(1):461.

5. Mazzaferri EL, Jhiang SM. Long-term impact of initial surgical and medical therapy on papillary and follicular thyroid cancer. Am J Med 1994;97(5):418–28.

6. Randolph GW, Duh QY, Heller KS, et al. The prognostic significance of nodal metastases from papillary thyroid carcinoma can be stratified based on the size and number of metastatic lymph nodes, as well as the presence of extranodal extension. Thyroid 2012;22(11):1144–52.

7. Adam MA, Pura J, Goffredo P, et al. Impact of extent of surgery on survival for papillary thyroid cancer patients younger than 45 years. J Clin Endocrinol Metab 2015;100(1):115–21.

8. American Joint Committee On C, Amin MB, Edge SB, et al. AJCC cancer staging Manual. Eighth edition. Springer; 2017. xvii, 1032 pages : illustrations (black and white, and colour).

9. Zaydfudim V, Feurer ID, Griffin MR, et al. The impact of lymph node involvement on survival in patients with papillary and follicular thyroid carcinoma. Surg 2008; 144(6):1070–7 [discussion: 1077-8].

10. Medas F, Canu GL, Boi F, et al. Predictive Factors of Recurrence in Patients with Differentiated Thyroid Carcinoma: A Retrospective Analysis on 579 Patients. Cancers (Basel) 2019;(9):11. https://doi.org/10.3390/cancers11091230.

11. Wang LY, Palmer FL, Nixon IJ, et al. Central lymph node characteristics predictive of outcome in patients with differentiated thyroid cancer. Thyroid 2014;24(12): 1790–5.

12. Haugen BR, Alexander EK, Bible KC, et al. 2015 American Thyroid Association Management Guidelines for Adult Patients with Thyroid Nodules and Differentiated Thyroid Cancer: The American Thyroid Association Guidelines Task Force on Thyroid Nodules and Differentiated Thyroid Cancer. Thyroid 2016;26(1):1–133.

13. Ramirez A, Sanabria A. Prophylactic central neck dissection for well-differentiated thyroid carcinoma: results and methodological assessment of systematic reviews. JBI Evid Synth 2022;20(4):980–1003.

14. Sturgeon C, Yang A, Elaraj D. Surgical Management of Lymph Node Compartments in Papillary Thyroid Cancer. Surg Oncol Clin N Am 2016;25(1):17–40.

15. Leboulleux S, Girard E, Rose M, et al. Ultrasound criteria of malignancy for cervical lymph nodes in patients followed up for differentiated thyroid cancer. J Clin Endocrinol Metab 2007;92(9):3590–4.

16. Zhao H, Li H. Meta-analysis of ultrasound for cervical lymph nodes in papillary thyroid cancer: Diagnosis of central and lateral compartment nodal metastases. Eur J Radiol 2019;112:14–21.

17. Roh JL, Kim JM, Park CI. Central lymph node metastasis of unilateral papillary thyroid carcinoma: patterns and factors predictive of nodal metastasis, morbidity, and recurrence. Ann Surg Oncol 2011;18(8):2245–50.

18. Al-Hilli Z, Strajina V, McKenzie TJ, et al. Thyroglobulin Measurement in Fine-Needle Aspiration Improves the Diagnosis of Cervical Lymph Node Metastases in Papillary Thyroid Carcinoma. Ann Surg Oncol 2017;24(3):739–44.

19. Xing Z, Qiu Y, Yang Q, et al. Thyroid cancer neck lymph nodes metastasis: Meta-analysis of US and CT diagnosis. Eur J Radiol 2020;129:109103.

20. Kim SK, Woo JW, Park I, et al. Computed Tomography-Detected Central Lymph Node Metastasis in Ultrasonography Node-Negative Papillary Thyroid Carcinoma: Is It Really Significant? Ann Surg Oncol 2017;24(2):442–9.
21. Scherl S, Mehra S, Clain J, et al. The effect of surgeon experience on the detection of metastatic lymph nodes in the central compartment and the pathologic features of clinically unapparent metastatic lymph nodes: what are we missing when we don't perform a prophylactic dissection of central compartment lymph nodes in papillary thyroid cancer? Thyroid 2014;24(8):1282–8.
22. Kim MJ, Kim HJ, Park CS, et al. Frozen section analysis of central lymph nodes in papillary thyroid cancer: the significance in determining the extent of surgery. Gland Surg 2022;11(4):640–50.
23. Shaha AR, Tuttle RM. Frozen section of central lymph nodes in thyroid cancer. Gland Surg 2022;11(4):637–9.
24. Albers MB, Nordenstrom E, Wohlfahrt J, et al. Sentinel Lymph Node Biopsy in Thyroid Cancer. World J Surg 2020;44(1):142–7.
25. Yan Y, Wang Y, Liu N, et al. Predictive value of the Delphian lymph node in cervical lymph node metastasis of papillary thyroid carcinoma. Eur J Surg Oncol 2021; 47(7):1727–33.
26. Jonker PKC, Metman MJH, Sondorp LHJ, et al. Intraoperative MET-receptor targeted fluorescent imaging and spectroscopy for lymph node detection in papillary thyroid cancer: novel diagnostic tools for more selective central lymph node compartment dissection. Eur J Nucl Med Mol Imaging 2022. https://doi.org/10.1007/s00259-022-05763-3.
27. American Thyroid Association Surgery Working G, American Association of Endocrine S, American Academy of O-H, et al. Consensus statement on the terminology and classification of central neck dissection for thyroid cancer. Thyroid 2009;19(11):1153–8.
28. Agrawal N, Evasovich MR, Kandil E, et al. Indications and extent of central neck dissection for papillary thyroid cancer: An American Head and Neck Society Consensus Statement. Head Neck 2017;39(7):1269–79.
29. Park YM, Lee SM, Kim DW, et al. Predictive factors of right paraesophageal lymph node metastasis in papillary thyroid carcinoma: Single center experience and meta-analysis. PLoS One 2017;12(5):e0177956.
30. Kim D, Kwon HK, Shin SC, et al. Right posterior paratracheal lymph nodes metastasis is one of the predictive factors in right-sided papillary thyroid carcinoma. Surgery 2019;166(6):1154–9.
31. Likhterov I, Reis LL, Urken ML. Central compartment management in patients with papillary thyroid cancer presenting with metastatic disease to the lateral neck: Anatomic pathways of lymphatic spread. Head Neck 2017;39(5):853–9.
32. Fraser S, Zaidi N, Norlen O, et al. Incidence and Risk Factors for Occult Level 3 Lymph Node Metastases in Papillary Thyroid Cancer. Ann Surg Oncol 2016; 23(11):3587–92.
33. Hu D, Lin H, Zeng X, et al. Risk Factors for and Prediction Model of Skip Metastasis to Lateral Lymph Nodes in Papillary Thyroid Carcinoma. World J Surg 2020; 44(5):1498–505.
34. Zhao H, Huang T, Li H. Risk factors for skip metastasis and lateral lymph node metastasis of papillary thyroid cancer. Surgery 2019;166(1):55–60.
35. Harries V, McGill M, Tuttle RM, et al. Management of Retropharyngeal Lymph Node Metastases in Differentiated Thyroid Carcinoma. Thyroid 2020;30(5): 688–95.

36. Feng JW, Qu Z, Ye J, et al. Nomograms to predict ipsilateral and contralateral central lymph node metastasis in clinically lymph node-negative patients with solitary isthmic classic papillary thyroid carcinoma. Surgery 2021;170(6):1670–9.

37. Song CM, Lee DW, Ji YB, et al. Frequency and pattern of central lymph node metastasis in papillary carcinoma of the thyroid isthmus. Head Neck 2016; 38(Suppl 1):E412–6.

38. Musacchio MJ, Kim AW, Vijungco JD, et al. Greater local recurrence occurs with "berry picking" than neck dissection in thyroid cancer. Am Surg 2003;69(3):191-6 ; discussion 196-7.

39. Kouvaraki MA, Lee JE, Shapiro SE, et al. Preventable reoperations for persistent and recurrent papillary thyroid carcinoma. Surgery 2004;136(6):1183–91.

40. Sun R, Sheng J, Zhou Y, et al. Relationship between the extent of central node dissection and parathyroid function preservation in thyroid cancer surgery. Gland Surg 2021;10(3):1093–103.

41. Wang LY, Versnick MA, Gill AJ, et al. Level VII is an important component of central neck dissection for papillary thyroid cancer. Ann Surg Oncol 2013;20(7): 2261–5.

42. Kim DH, Kim SW, Hwang SH. Predictive Value of Delphian Lymph Node Metastasis in the Thyroid Cancer. Laryngoscope 2021;131(9):1990–6.

43. Isaacs JD, Lundgren CI, Sidhu SB, et al. The Delphian lymph node in thyroid cancer. Ann Surg 2008;247(3):477–82.

44. Kaul P, Kaul P, Poonia DR, et al. Risk Benefit Analysis of Routine Thymectomy for Differentiated Thyroid Cancers: A Systematic Review. Surg J (N Y) 2021;7(4): e307–13.

45. Robinson TJ, Thomas S, Dinan MA, et al. How Many Lymph Nodes Are Enough? Assessing the Adequacy of Lymph Node Yield for Papillary Thyroid Cancer. J Clin Oncol 2016;34(28):3434–9.

46. Medas F, Canu GL, Cappellacci F, et al. Prophylactic Central Lymph Node Dissection Improves Disease-Free Survival in Patients with Intermediate and High Risk Differentiated Thyroid Carcinoma: A Retrospective Analysis on 399 Patients. Cancers (Basel) 2020;(6):12. https://doi.org/10.3390/cancers12061658.

47. Chen L, Wu YH, Lee CH, et al. Prophylactic Central Neck Dissection for Papillary Thyroid Carcinoma with Clinically Uninvolved Central Neck Lymph Nodes: A Systematic Review and Meta-analysis. World J Surg 2018;42(9):2846–57.

48. Zhao WJ, Luo H, Zhou YM, et al. Evaluating the effectiveness of prophylactic central neck dissection with total thyroidectomy for cN0 papillary thyroid carcinoma: An updated meta-analysis. Eur J Surg Oncol 2017;43(11):1989–2000.

49. Alsubaie KM, Alsubaie HM, Alzahrani FR, et al. Prophylactic Central Neck Dissection for Clinically Node-Negative Papillary Thyroid Carcinoma. Laryngoscope 2021.

50. Sippel RS, Robbins SE, Poehls JL, et al. A Randomized Controlled Clinical Trial: No Clear Benefit to Prophylactic Central Neck Dissection in Patients With Clinically Node Negative Papillary Thyroid Cancer. Ann Surg 2020;272(3):496–503.

51. Sanabria A, Betancourt C, Sanchez JG, et al. Prophylactic Central Neck Lymph Node Dissection in Low-Risk Thyroid Carcinoma Patients Does not Decrease the Incidence of Locoregional Recurrence: A Meta-Analysis of Randomized Trials. Ann Surg 2022.

52. Ahn JH, Kwak JH, Yoon SG, et al. A prospective randomized controlled trial to assess the efficacy and safety of prophylactic central compartment lymph node dissection in papillary thyroid carcinoma. Surg 2022;171(1):182–9.

53. Wang TS, Cheung K, Farrokhyar F, et al. A meta-analysis of the effect of prophylactic central compartment neck dissection on locoregional recurrence rates in patients with papillary thyroid cancer. Ann Surg Oncol 2013;20(11):3477–83.
54. Jo YJ, Choi HR, Park SH, et al. Extent of thyroid surgery for clinically node-negative papillary thyroid carcinoma with confirmed nodal metastases after prophylactic central neck dissection: a 15-year experience in a single center. Ann Surg Treat Res 2020;99(4):197–204.
55. Nylen C, Eriksson FB, Yang A, et al. Prophylactic central lymph node dissection informs the decision of radioactive iodine ablation in papillary thyroid cancer. Am J Surg 2021;221(5):886–92.
56. Hughes DT, Rosen JE, Evans DB, et al. Prophylactic Central Compartment Neck Dissection in Papillary Thyroid Cancer and Effect on Locoregional Recurrence. Ann Surg Oncol 2018;25(9):2526–34.
57. Sawka AM, Brierley JD, Tsang RW, et al. An updated systematic review and commentary examining the effectiveness of radioactive iodine remnant ablation in well-differentiated thyroid cancer. Endocrinol Metab Clin North Am 2008;37(2):457–80, x.
58. McHenry CR. Is Prophylactic Central Compartment Neck Dissection Indicated for Clinically Node-Negative Papillary Thyroid Cancer: The Answer is Dependent on How the Data are Interpreted and the Weight Given to the Risks and Benefits. Ann Surg Oncol 2018;25(11):3123–4.
59. Viola D, Materazzi G, Valerio L, et al. Prophylactic central compartment lymph node dissection in papillary thyroid carcinoma: clinical implications derived from the first prospective randomized controlled single institution study. J Clin Endocrinol Metab 2015;100(4):1316–24.
60. Filetti S, Durante C, Hartl D, et al. Thyroid cancer: ESMO Clinical Practice Guidelines for diagnosis, treatment and follow-updagger. Ann Oncol 2019;30(12):1856–83.
61. Sywak M, Cornford L, Roach P, et al. Routine ipsilateral level VI lymphadenectomy reduces postoperative thyroglobulin levels in papillary thyroid cancer. Surgery 2006;140(6):1000–5 [discussion: 1005-7].
62. Korkmaz MH, Ocal B, Saylam G, et al. The need of prophylactic central lymph node dissection is controversial in terms of postoperative thyroglobulin follow-up of patients with cN0 papillary thyroid cancer. Langenbecks Arch Surg 2017;402(2):235–42.
63. Medas F, Tuveri M, Canu GL, et al. Complications after reoperative thyroid surgery: retrospective evaluation of 152 consecutive cases. Updates Surg 2019;71(4):705–10.
64. Alvarado R, Sywak MS, Delbridge L, et al. Central lymph node dissection as a secondary procedure for papillary thyroid cancer: Is there added morbidity? Surgery 2009;145(5):514–8.
65. Lombardi D, Accorona R, Paderno A, et al. Morbidity of central neck dissection for papillary thyroid cancer. Gland Surg 2017;6(5):492–500.
66. Selberherr A, Riss P, Scheuba C, et al. Prophylactic "First-Step" Central Neck Dissection (Level 6) Does Not Increase Morbidity After (Total) Thyroidectomy. Ann Surg Oncol 2016;23(12):4016–22.
67. Mitchell AL, Gandhi A, Scott-Coombes D, et al. Management of thyroid cancer: United Kingdom National Multidisciplinary Guidelines. J Laryngol Otol 2016;130(S2):S150–60.
68. NCCN) NCCN. Thyroid carcinoma: NCCN clinical Practice guidelines in Oncology (NCCN Guidelines®). 2022. Available at: https://www.nccn.org/

professionals/physician_gls/pdf/thyroid.pdf. Updated Version 2.2022 — May 5, 2022. Accessed 23 06 2022.

69. Ito Y, Onoda N, Okamoto T. The revised clinical practice guidelines on the management of thyroid tumors by the Japan Associations of Endocrine Surgeons: Core questions and recommendations for treatments of thyroid cancer. Endocr J 2020;67(7):669–717.

70. Sancho JJ, Lennard TW, Paunovic I, et al. Prophylactic central neck disection in papillary thyroid cancer: a consensus report of the European Society of Endocrine Surgeons (ESES). Langenbecks Arch Surg 2014;399(2):155–63.

71. Ma B, Wang Y, Yang S, et al. Predictive factors for central lymph node metastasis in patients with cN0 papillary thyroid carcinoma: A systematic review and meta-analysis. Int J Surg 2016;28:153–61.

72. Carling T, Carty SE, Ciarleglio MM, et al. American Thyroid Association design and feasibility of a prospective randomized controlled trial of prophylactic central lymph node dissection for papillary thyroid carcinoma. Thyroid 2012;22(3):237–44.

73. Sutherland R, Tsang V, Clifton-Bligh RJ, et al. Papillary thyroid microcarcinoma: Is active surveillance always enough? Clin Endocrinol (Oxf) 2021;95(6):811–7.

74. Papachristos AJ, Do K, Tsang V, et al. Outcomes of papillary thyroid microcarcinoma presenting with palpable lateral lymphadenopathy. Thyroid 2022.

75. Wen X, Jin Q, Cen X, et al. Clinicopathologic predictors of central lymph node metastases in clinical node-negative papillary thyroid microcarcinoma: a systematic review and meta-analysis. World J Surg Oncol 2022;20(1):106.

76. Ryu YJ, Yoon JH. Impact of prophylactic unilateral central neck dissection needed for patients with papillary thyroid microcarcinoma. Gland Surg 2020;9(2):352–61.

77. Yan XQ, Zhang ZZ, Yu WJ, et al. Prophylactic Central Neck Dissection for cN1b Papillary Thyroid Carcinoma: A Systematic Review and Meta-Analysis. Front Oncol 2021;11:803986.

78. Harries V, McGill M, Wang LY, et al. Is a Prophylactic Central Compartment Neck Dissection Required in Papillary Thyroid Carcinoma Patients with Clinically Involved Lateral Compartment Lymph Nodes? Ann Surg Oncol 2021;28(1):512–8.

79. Carmel-Neiderman NN, Mizrachi A, Yaniv D, et al. Prophylactic central neck dissection has no advantage in patients with metastatic papillary thyroid cancer to the lateral neck. J Surg Oncol 2021;123(2):456–61.

80. De Napoli L, Matrone A, Favilla K, et al. Role of Prophylactic Central Compartment Lymph Node Dissection on the Outcome Of Patients With Papillary Thyroid Carcinoma and Synchronous Ipsilateral Cervical Lymph Node Metastases. Endocr Pract 2020;26(8):807–17.

81. Zatelli MC, Lamartina L, Meringolo D, et al. Thyroid nodule recurrence following lobo-isthmectomy: incidence, patient's characteristics, and risk factors. J Endocrinol Invest 2018;41(12):1469–75.

82. Grani G, Lamartina L, Durante C, et al. Follicular thyroid cancer and Hurthle cell carcinoma: challenges in diagnosis, treatment, and clinical management. Lancet Diabetes Endocrinol 2018;6(6):500–14.

83. Perros P, Boelaert K, Colley S, et al. Guidelines for the management of thyroid cancer. Clin Endocrinol (Oxf) 2014;81(Suppl 1):1–122.